# LIVING WITH
# ARTHRITIS

## PEOPLE WITH ARTHRITIS TALK
## ABOUT COPING FROM DAY TO DAY

*PUBLISHED IN ASSOCIATION WITH ARTHRITIS CARE*

## Michael Leitch

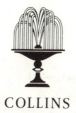

COLLINS

## ACKNOWLEDGEMENTS

The author would like to thank the twenty-seven contributors who kindly agreed to talk to him about their experiences of arthritis. Thanks are also due to Carol Holland of Arthritis Care for her considerable help and advice during the preparation of this book.

First published in 1987 by
William Collins Sons & Co., Ltd
London · Glasgow · Sydney · Auckland · Toronto ·
Johannesburg

© Lennard Books 1987

**British Library Cataloguing in Publication Data**

Living with arthritis.
1. Rheumatoid arthritis – Psychological aspects
I. Michael Leitch
362.1′96722    RC933

ISBN 0 00 218244 0

Set in Crown
by V & M Graphics Ltd, Aylesbury, Bucks
Printed and bound in Great Britain
by Robert Hartnoll (1985) Ltd, Bodmin

# CONTENTS

# FOREWORD

## Terry Wogan

Let me get the main plug in early. *Everybody* should read this book. Not that everybody doesn't know about arthritis – they *must* do. There are upwards of *8 million* sufferers from the disease, in its various forms, in Great Britain; around one in seven of the population. Few other diseases, if any, ever make such a claim to national popularity. Or, more correctly, unpopularity. Everybody in these islands knows somebody with arthritis: friends, neighbours, relatives ....

You wouldn't think it necessary, therefore, to have to bawl continually from the rooftops to draw the public's attention to this crippling, awful disease, that affects so grievously the lives of so many of their loved ones. But, believe me, a pretty continuous roar has to be kept up before anyone casts more than a mildly interested glance in the direction of arthritis.

Mention cancer, lifeboats, sick and indigent room-keepers, the Donkey Sanctuary, and you have people dabbing at their eyes with one hand, and reaching for their chequebooks with the other. Now, I've nothing against donkeys – some of my best friends in television criticism bear more than a passing resemblance to the noble animals, and in that 'far, fierce hour and sweet' in Jerusalem, Christ Himself rode a donkey – but when people leave more money in their wills to the sanctuary of donkeys than they do to Arthritis Care, then I think some of us can be pardoned for gnawing the wainscoting ....

Perhaps it's because the disease is so common that it provokes such a nonplussed reaction. The heart and nervous diseases, and, of course, cancer, seem to engender an

4

emotional response from the public; arthritis has all the emotional impact of a blancmange. The public's perception of arthritis is of a painful, but harmless disease that never killed anybody. Cancer kills, heart disease kills, but arthritis? It's old people in wheelchairs, isn't it?

Well, yes, it does, and no, it isn't. Arthritis kills in the worst way: by attrition. Slowly, painfully, eating away at the body until the spirit is broken, and the very will to live is gone. It may take twenty, thirty, forty years but, believe me, in its own way arthritis can kill. Old people in wheelchairs? Yes, plenty of them – *millions*. But *young* people in wheelchairs, too. Even babies can develop arthritis. Walk into a ward full of little children suffering from arthritis, and *then* tell me about a disease that provokes an emotional response.

Every year, in one of the less grand London hotels, it's my privilege and honour to present the 'Dista' awards to young people with arthritis who, by dint of courage, intelligence and determination, have overcome physical handicap, pain, and what to most people would be insurmountable difficulty, to achieve their goals. To give an example of the calibre of these people: a couple of years ago, one of the winners was a girl of nineteen. Arthritis had confined her to a wheelchair for most of her life, left her with a body that could do virtually nothing for itself, and blinded her. Yet, she had won a place at university! The brain was working perfectly, you see, and the spirit was unquenchable. It's difficult not to weep with pity and admiration in the presence of such people, but they don't feel sorry for themselves, so why should you? They present an indomitable, optimistic face to the world, and they don't want your pity. They don't even ask for your support. But I do.

Read this book. It's full to bursting with good practical advice from people with arthritis on how to cope with the disease in all its forms. This is an invaluable handbook for arthritis sufferers, their families, friends and helpers, on how to deal with almost every aspect of everyday living, both private and public, from the kitchen to the supermarket, from the wheelchair to the bus. In here, you'll find articles from people with arthritis in every walk of life: from the television presenter David Icke and the journalist Marje Proops, to the MP Jo Richardson and the typist David Webb. What you'll find here, too, is what you find in profusion in all people with arthritis: courage.

I became involved with Arthritis Care for personal rather than altruistic reasons: my mother has suffered badly from rheumatoid arthritis for at least twenty-five years. An active and vital woman cut down in her prime, who has endured constant pain, discomfiture and numerous operations to hands and legs. She's still smiling, she's still cheerful, but there's probably little hope of a cure for her. All we can do is ease the pain, help the mobility, and respond to her marvellous personality with an equally cheerful face.

There's somebody *you* know out there with arthritis. They won't ask for your help. They may not even look like they need it. They do. We *all* do, if we're going to win the battle against arthritis. Help, if you can. Start here.

Terry Wogan
Chairman of Arthritis Care's Appeals and
Public Relations Committee

6

# AUTHOR'S NOTE

This book presents a multiple view of what it is like to have arthritis. It is mainly compiled from a collection of interviews with twenty-seven contributors who, with great frankness and generosity, and not a little humour, talked about how the disease affects them and how they cope with it in their daily lives.

If they were all to meet in a room, not only would the noise be deafening, it is unlikely they would all agree with each other. That is hardly surprising, since arthritis is a disease of many different aspects. One description of it may seem to contradict another, though both are true. What is more, arthritis claims its sufferers from every age group, social condition and outlook. The views of the contributors are very much their own and do not necessarily coincide with those of Arthritis Care, the organization to which many of them, though not all, belong and which has been responsible for developing this book.

It should also be stressed that this is not a medical book. (The medical viewpoint can be found in some of the publications listed at the end of the book.) Many hints and helpful suggestions are offered with a view to increasing awareness of the disease and making home and family life easier. These are intended to encourage a spirit of independence, but are in no way a substitute for medical aid. The first person to go to for medical advice is, as ever, the family doctor, and all subsequent consultations and treatment should stem from him.

Those ground rules stated, we hope this book will be both helpful and stimulating. If the contributors share one attitude, it is that life is more important than arthritis.

# FACTS ABOUT ARTHRITIS

Arthritis is a common complaint. In Britain as many as 20 million people experience some form of rheumatic complaint during the course of a year, and more than 8 million consult their doctor about it.

While it is true that arthritis occurs most frequently among the elderly, it is not true that arthritis is a disease that only old people can get. Arthritis affects all ages. Even children may suffer from it: currently about 15,000 children in Britain have a juvenile form of arthritis.

There are some typical sufferers. Rheumatoid arthritis affects three times as many women as men, and the typical sufferer is a woman in her thirties or over. Ankylosing spondylitis, which affects the joints of the spine and pelvis, tends to occur in young men in their late teens and early twenties. Osteoarthritis usually affects people from about the age of fifty. Few people over the age of sixty remain free of arthritis for the rest of their lives.

## What is Arthritis?

To medical people the word arthritis means specifically inflammation of the joints, from the Greek *arthron* (joint) and *-itis* (inflammation). Today it has a more popular meaning which covers the rheumatic diseases in general and thus embraces all forms of pain in the bones, muscles, joints and tissues which surround the joints. This is the meaning used in the book.

There are some two hundred types of arthritis. Sufferers develop individual problems, and treatments are varied to suit each case. The two hundred types fall into the following principal groups: osteoarthritis; rheumatoid arthritis; gout; ankylosing spondylitis; other types, including arthritis associated with lupus; and various forms of soft-tissue rheumatism (e.g. bad shoulders).

### Osteoarthritis

This is also, and more correctly, known as osteoarthrosis, since it is not an inflammatory disease, but one which produces damage in the joints. It is the most common form of arthritis; in

Britain about five million people suffer from it. One in six people consulting their doctor about a rheumatic complaint is found to have osteoarthritis.

It is caused by a wearing away of the cartilage at the end of the bones. The surface of the cartilage becomes roughened and in places splits; the underlying bone then thickens and grows outwards, enlarging the joint. Surrounding the bone ends and the cartilage is a lining called the synovium. This may become inflamed and the extra fluid that forms makes the joint swell.

The most commonly affected joints are the hips, knees, spine, hands and feet. Osteoarthritis usually begins in one joint, which becomes stiff and painful, and may then spread to other joints. In severe cases the joints become deformed, restricting movement.

## Rheumatoid arthritis

This is a fairly common disease, affecting one out of thirty people consulting their doctor about a rheumatic complaint – about half a million in Britain. It is a systemic disease; it causes inflammation of the joint lining and swelling in the joints, and can be severely disabling.

The most commonly affected joints are the hands, wrists, elbows, shoulders, knees and feet. Painful swelling may occur over a period of days or weeks, or suddenly in a matter of hours. Morning stiffness is characteristic. As well as feeling local pain, sufferers may feel generally unwell; there may be anaemia, fatigue and weight loss. The disease may follow a pattern in which active flare-ups are followed by periods of remission or respite.

## Gout

Gout usually causes a single joint to become inflamed, producing a very sharp tormenting pain. Acute gouty arthritis is caused by crystals of sodium urate entering a joint and provoking a reaction in the tissue. The affected joint swells, turns bluish-red and shiny, and is extremely tender. It is much more common in men than women (seven to one or more).

The most commonly affected joints are the big toes (more than 70 per cent of cases), feet, ankles, knees, fingers and wrists. Acute gouty arthritis can be effectively controlled by drugs, and may either occur only once or twice in the sufferer's lifetime, or with increasing severity, perhaps entering a chronic secondary stage.

## Ankylosing spondylitis

This is an inflammatory disease of the spinal joints which usually affects young men. It is sometimes known as 'poker back' or 'bamboo spine' because in developed cases there are bony outgrowths and the vertebrae may become fused. The larger joints of the body may be affected as well. It can also affect the eyes – in fact, it may start with eye problems.

## Lupus

This is a rheumatic disease about which little was known before 1948. Its full name is systemic lupus erythematosus (SLE). It is caused by an upset to the body's immune system. The sufferer produces an excess of antibodies (blood proteins), which circulate and cause problems in one or more areas, including the skin, the kidney, the heart and lungs, and the joints; more rarely the brain may be affected. Lupus is much more common in women than men (about nine to one), and typically appears in young women in their teens and twenties.

Lupus may show itself in the form of a facial rash and is named after the group of 'wolf' rashes – the term used by physicians in former times to describe rashes on the cheeks and nose; most typical of these is the butterfly-shaped rash. The disease may begin slowly or acutely. There may be fever, fatigue, headaches, and muscle and joint pains. Exposure to sunlight may cause a flare-up; there may be hair loss, inflammation of the tendons or of the veins and arteries. For most sufferers, however, the disease is concentrated in one organ or system of the body.

## What to Do

The trouble with descriptions of diseases is that they tend to give you a lot of facts in one large, unwelcome, possibly frightening lump. Before we go any further it is important to emphasize that people can suffer from some forms of arthritis without feeling pain or ever needing to consult their doctor. Others may suffer so mildly that the disease makes only a shallow intrusion into their lives.

For people whose arthritis gives them more than occasional discomfort, the picture need not be as bleak as it may once have seemed. Many children, for example, now make a full recovery from juvenile arthritis and are able to look forward to a normal adult life. Effective treatments now exist for some rheumatic diseases, such as gout, and great steps have been taken in recent years to relieve the pain and suffering associated with all the rheumatic diseases. Much more research needs to be done into the causes of many of them, and at present no cures have yet been found. In the meantime, however, there is much that the sufferer can do to make life easier and better.

The first rule must be this: if you suffer persistent pain in one or more joints, go and see your family doctor. He should always be your first contact. What happens next will depend on what kind of arthritis you appear to have and how much of a problem it is. You may be referred to a rheumatologist, a specialist doctor at a hospital, for further advice and treatment.

Therapists are also available to help you. Exercise is both beneficial and necessary in the treatment of many rheumatic diseases, and physiotherapists can do a lot to keep their patients moving – by increasing the strength of their muscles and by improving the range of movement in their joints and limbs.

Occupational therapists provide another kind of service. They advise on how to look after the joints in daily life. They can provide aids and appliances, for example, and recommend major improvements such as a redesigned kitchen or bathroom.

Then, of course, there is you, and the things you can do for yourself. Coping with arthritis can be hard work at times, but most efforts bring a reward, moving the sufferer towards new levels of understanding and ability. The purpose of the chapters that follow is to demonstrate some of the many options that are now available for anyone with a mind to pursue them.

# ONE MAN'S SAGA

## The Lord Killearn

---

No single account of the onset of arthritis and its treatment can be typical for all, but this description by Lord Killearn contains many elements that sufferers will recognize. In a sense he has experienced an Arthritic Saga which falls into two distinct parts. Fortunately, and thanks to the excellent treatment he has received, Part II has turned out a great deal better for him than Part I.

---

## Part I: The First Eleven Years

The story begins in about 1975, when I was in my middle fifties and developed an intensely painful back. I felt all sorts of curious, unpredictable pains shooting down my legs. It felt as if these pains were in the sciatic nerves, but they were not. The trouble was in the lower back, where the bones were out of position and pressing on a nerve, and the pain was being referred down the legs. This condition was occasioned, I believe, by a skiing fall: in about 1958 I was knocked out for a couple of days, but thereafter felt perfectly OK again.

In 1977 I fell off a step-ladder, while pruning a rose or something equally stupid. This produced quite a bit of pain in my left knee where I had torn a ligament about ten years previously (also skiing). I subsequently began to have trouble with my right knee, which later gave me more pain than anything else. I think that was because I had overloaded it.

To return to my back, which originally was the worst thing but subsequently became the least, my then doctor was excellent. He advised a very simple and drastic treatment. This consisted of resting absolutely still for a few days; putting a hard board under my mattress; losing weight; and swimming.

I did the first of these, and I did lose some weight – if not perhaps as much as my doctor would have liked. When it came to swimming, my initial problem was finding somewhere to do it. I found a public baths within 500 yds (450 m) of my office, which seemed fine. I then discovered that I could not walk 500 yds (450 m). I would get about halfway and then fold up, looking sometimes as if violently drunk!

This deterred me from going to swimming pools. Fortunately, my doctor took a firm line and insisted that I carry on. 'You really must swim,' he said. 'It's essential!'

I searched some more, and found a pool I could get close to by car. Once in the water, my very first strokes made the most fantastic difference – so much so that I felt as if I had been restored to normal. I still had some stiffness but, in general, I didn't feel too much pain.

Over the years, however, I slowly got worse. I tried a number of remedies, including courses of physiotherapy, hydrotherapy, zone therapy (also known as reflexology), and osteopathy. Looking back, my feeling is that these treatments only kept me at a certain level: I had delayed the process of degeneration but not halted it.

The main problem I had was not so much bending my knees as getting them to straighten. One knee was fifteen degrees out of line, the other five degrees; this made walking and, particularly, standing very difficult.

I should add that over those last few years I had had several medical checks with hospital consultants, x-rays and blood tests, so I was not merely carrying out a series of personal forays into fringe medicine. I had also kept in close touch with the medical establishment.

Another problem I developed was swollen legs. The first attack, in 1980, came on suddenly and in a matter of hours I had a high temperature and a right ankle which had developed a painful lymphatic 'boil'. With antibiotics it then subsided almost as rapidly. In 1982 and 1983 I had a second, much slower, less feverish attack in the left leg and foot. This took a long time to come up but it swelled enormously and grew very hot and tender before eventually peeling. Although there was no direct connection between either of these problems and my arthritic condition, they certainly did not help. The swellings largely went down, but not entirely in the left leg.

During the course of 1985, when I thought I really was not going to get much better in a hurry, I went to see a surgeon about my knees. He suggested that it would be a good idea if I had my knees operated on, adding that artificial knees were now very good. 'It will certainly relieve the pain,' he said, 'and help you to stand straighter.'

Everything seemed to be in favour of my having the operations. I felt rather pleased; the idea of bringing these problems to a head at last was something that appealed to me. My wife, however, reminded me that I was overweight, had a circulation problem, and was no longer young. I should not be too light-hearted about putting myself into hospital for two quite major operations.

I agreed to seek a second opinion. We went to see another surgeon and he endorsed her doubts. He took one look at me and declared that he would not consider taking me on.

'You're far too heavy,' he said. 'You need to lose 4 st ((25 kg). *And* you have a circulation problem. In any case,' he went on, 'even if you came back in six months, having lost all that weight, and with good circulation, I would still very likely say no.'

The reason was that although he was perfectly confident about hip operations, which were comparatively simple to carry out with prostheses that now lasted for ten to fifteen years, knee replacements were much less certain. 'I could not guarantee that there would be no complications or pain,' he said. 'The knee is a very difficult joint.'

So there I was. My wife and I were both in a sense relieved, but I had not advanced my position at all. It was at about this time that I opted to use two sticks.

I had been using one stick for some time, but because lack of balance was a greater problem than flexibility or strength, I decided two would be better. When going up or down stairs or steps, I was quite happy if I had a wall to lean a hand on or a rail to grasp; but in the middle of a broad flight of steps, without lateral support, I was lost.

When we moved into our present house some fifteen years ago, we thought how easy and convenient it was compared with our previous rather larger home: fewer rooms, fewer stairs – we were sure it would suit us better. In recent years, however, it seemed to grow bigger each year, and the stairs steeper!

I was now, in fact, finding that stairs required quite an effort – and so was my wife, for different reasons. Inevitably one is faced with a lot of lifting and carrying in the course of an ordinary day. Now, however, I could not manage to carry a tray from one floor to another. Fairly recently, therefore, we decided to sell the house and move into a flat, and this we are in the process of doing.

My life became restricted in other ways, too. If we were invited to a party which might involve a lot of standing, I would not go. I also felt embarrassed about not getting up for people, and that sort of thing. I had firmly set my mind against going into a wheelchair, however, if I could possibly avoid it, although on some occasions – at airports, for instance – I didn't mind being pushed about. At Gatwick they lay on an electric buggy for you, which is splendid. I didn't mind that at all but, in general, I still rejected the idea of a permanent wheelchair.

I had also cut down on some of my work in the House of Lords. I had been on a number of parliamentary visits – to Syria, Romania, the United States – each of which took several days. Hitherto I had not held up things too much: now I decided that I really was too slow and should not try to carry on.

The same applied to Services visits, at home or abroad. Hopping in and out of an armoured car or even a bus, and going up and down companionways on board ship became a problem; I was now not mobile enough to get around properly. At one point, when contemplating going to watch some BAOR (British Army of the Rhine) exercises, I was told by a friendly contact at the Ministry of Defence: 'Look, for your own good, I don't think you will enjoy this. It will be very strenuous and you will run the risk of holding up others.'

So, one way and another, I became resigned to the fact that I had to lead my life in a lower gear. I could still stand about if I had to, though I found walking easier – as a lot of people with knee trouble do. Even so, I didn't like walking far, not more than 200 yds (180 m) at most. I had developed drills for various things like getting in and out of cars and taxis. Fortunately I was able to drive quite happily. Provided the weight was off my knees – when I was lying, sitting or driving – I had very little pain.

That was the story of my arthritis until the end of July 1986. I had adapted to living more slowly, and hoped that I could continue on that basis indefinitely: in a flat, on two sticks, and without a chair.

# Part II: All Change

Then, within a few days, I suddenly found myself in hospital and receiving special treatment of a very different kind. I had woken one morning with a painful right shoulder. The pain spread to my neck, and after three days or so I had pain and stiffness in both shoulders, in my ribcage and waist; and my left hand and arm were very swollen and painful to the touch. Soon I was hardly able to move, not even to hump myself sideways along the edge of my bed.

I went into hospital where I was seen by a consultant rheumatologist. A blood sample was taken, which revealed a high ESR count – in other words, a high content of crystals in my blood. My general condition was diagnosed as acute polymyalgia rheumatica. The treatment consisted of several courses of tablets, including some steroids, running in parallel. These worked wonders: in two and a half weeks the ESR count was reduced to well within acceptable limits. At the same time I began attempts to re-establish my mobility: first with a frame, then walking with my own two sticks, then with an intensive course of exercises in the hydrotherapy pool.

As soon as it became evident that the tablets were being effective in cleaning up my blood, the consultant said he would like me to come back to the hospital after a suitable interval to have both knees 're-lined'. I should add that, shortly after my arrival in hospital, I had been put on a very strict diet. Each day I had a normal breakfast, but after that only orange juice was allowed – and in limited quantities. This regime and the strenuous exercise in the hydrotherapy pool combined to produce a weight reduction of some 2 st (13 kg) over the eighteen days I spent in hospital. I came out weighing about 14½ st (92 kg) – 4 st (25 kg) less than when I had seen the second surgeon the previous year!

At home I spent six and a half weeks pottering and generally regaining strength and confidence, but with no definite programme of exercise. I went for occasional hydrotherapy treatment and continued my 'starvation' diet.

When I reported back to the hospital my weight was 13½ st (86 kg). I marked time for a week while my blood count and general condition were given a final check. The operations were then done, and both have been resounding successes. I suffered no pain or ill effects. The prostheses are made of plastic and various non-ferrous alloys, and each knee weighs about 1½ lb (0.7 kg) more than my own knee did before, but to me this is not noticeable.

When I came out of hospital, five and a half months had gone by since my treatment for polymyalgia rheumatica had begun. I was by now fairly mobile, and both knees were able to bend to about ninety degrees. Although I was still, for safety, using two sticks, in fact I was able to manage with one and already felt that I might soon be able to dispense with even that.

It has been a remarkable sequence of events. I can now look forward to a relatively normal, mobile way of living – something that had seemed entirely out of the question for many years.

# ARTHRITIS IN THE HOME

## INTRODUCTION

Living with arthritis is a process of adapting to the changes in what we are able to do. The home is a natural starting point for this: the place in which we feel safe, warm and comfortable. That is, we *should* feel safe, warm and comfortable there, but probably only after we have done something about the stairs, found a suitable armchair, redesigned the bathroom, moved all the power points up the wall, bought a microwave....

You can, of course, go on for ever. That applies to able-bodied people, too. What we have tried to do in this section of the book is to round up some of the more typical problems affecting the daily home life of people with arthritis. There are seven chapters, in which contributors discuss mobility around the home; kitchen matters and shopping; adapting the bathroom, plus a few personal improvisations; coping from a wheelchair; coping from bed; a plea for more understanding by builders and others who instal things in our homes; and, finally, some ideas on how to set up your home in readiness for the day you come out of hospital after an operation.

In each of the first three chapters there is also a list of the many aids that can now make life easier around the home. These lists were compiled with the help of the Disabled Living Foundation and are based on the items exhibited at their Aids Centre in London. For further information on these and other home aids, including a list of regional aids centres, see the 'Help' section at the end of the book.

# KEEP MOVING

## Laura Mitchell

Laura Mitchell, MCSP, Dip TP, is a respected physiotherapist
and author, and a regular contributor to Central TV's *Getting
On* programme. She is familiar with arthritis from both inside
and out, having treated many arthritic patients while herself
suffering from osteoarthritis. She has undergone two hip
replacement operations, one of which did not work. Here she
talks about the problems of mobility around the home which
have affected her, and offers other suggestions for making life
better, safer and more comfortable.

Even as a small child I must have had a tendency towards
osteoarthritis, although it was never called that. I was always
being told to sit up straight. 'Your back's like a round O' was one
expression I remember. Yes, but I *couldn't* sit up straight. It was
too difficult. I could hold it for a while, but then I had to come
down again.

I hated gym, because I could not do things that the others did.
I could not touch my toes. Now I can, easily, and I am eighty, so
I must have had inflammation in the spine when I was young;
and that must have laid the foundation for the arthritis I
contracted later.

Ten years ago I had my first hip operation. This type of
operation was in its fairly early days then and unfortunately it
went wrong. It was all right for six months, then one morning I
got out of bed and nearly fell flat on my face. No-one could be
sure what my trouble was. They didn't know whether I was
allergic to the cement, or whether the thing was moving,
actually wobbling inside the joint. Meanwhile the pain became
intense, and I had to measure carefully what I could do without
making it worse. I was still working, going out in the car to see
patients, and did not wish to stop doing this as I still had to earn
my living.

It was at that stage that I rearranged my flat to suit my new limitations. In the kitchen, for instance, I arranged everything so that I could sit on my stool and make myself a cup of tea or coffee without getting up and moving about. The ingredients were all within easy reach, as well as the mugs, the kettle, everything. On another part of the work-top, I could bring up the stool, prepare vegetables and put them in a pan, slide the unwanted leaves, shells or other rubbish onto an old phone book and tip it into the rubbish bag which was underneath – all while sitting in the same place. I had another place where I ate, and by having these various centres of activity I saved myself a great deal of walking about.

There is another side to making your life easier, and that has to do with other people. I well remember sitting in my armchair and thinking that I would love a cup of tea, then deciding that it was not worth the pain of going and getting it. I wasn't too bad if I just sat still, so I'd stay where I was and go without the cup of tea.

I solved this problem by ringing a dear friend called Agnes who lived a few houses away. I found I could phone Agnes and say, 'Do you know anyone who makes cups of tea?' 'I'll be down in a minute,' she would always say – *dear* thing. And down she would come at any time to make me a cup of tea.

Having people around you who understand is just as important as rearranging things in the house. You don't want to become dependent on them, of course, but you do want people to help you – and for them to appreciate that you won't take advantage of them.

What I needed to do, I learned, was to find out what people enjoyed doing. For example, there was another woman I knew who loved shopping. 'Oh,' she said to me one day, 'I love spending other people's money!' So she took on my shopping for me. It did her good, too, I am sure. To go into a shop and say, 'I'll have that, that and that' made her feel quite powerful, especially when someone else was paying.

I am a person who must have silence about me for some of the time. If you are like me, beware the helper who *has* to talk, because they will use you as a pair of ears. They will stand about for half an hour after they have done what they came to do, and talk. In my experience none of this outpouring is worth hearing, but there is very little you can do about it if you can barely move. At the end of the half hour you are exhausted.

I do not wish to sound unappreciative, but the disabled have to look out for themselves. Just because you can't move easily doesn't mean that you are not still a living, breathing personality with your own set of desires. The worst thing of all is to give up and become a bundle.

## Sticks and Crutches

The first thing about sticks (and crutches) is that they must be the right height for you. There is an awful tendency to use 'Uncle George's stick' – that is, any old stick. People feel unsafe so they get themselves a third leg, but what they should do is get their *own* equipment through a physiotherapist.

The length of the stick should be determined by the distance from your wrist to the ground when your elbow is at an angle of about 135 degrees. If the stick is too short, you will injure your back as you lean forward; if it is too long, you will put your shoulder out. Make sure that every stick has a rubber ferrule on the end of it, and that the ferrule is replaced as soon as it gets worn.

The second thing about sticks (and crutches) is that you have to be taught how to use them. When they have acquired their third leg, many people tend to use it as exactly that. They fall into a rhythm of stick-leg-leg, stick-leg-leg, like a three-legged animal. If they have two sticks, it's worse. They either walk like a four-legged animal or they put two legs forward and bring up the other two behind.

Walking successfully with a stick bears little relation to normal walking. It has a different rhythm. The stick should be held in the opposite hand and placed exactly opposite the affected leg it is meant to support. Press down on the stick, stretch your back up, and walk with a normal gait. In this way you will still have, in your brain, a two-legged walk, now assisted by one or more sticks. Try also to be as upright as possible when you walk. Take comfort from the fact that it takes a baby about two years to learn a two-legged walk; make sure you don't lose the habit. Once they have lost it, many people find that they never go back to it.

In my own case, I have poor balance. On one side I have an artificial hip and on the other no hip at all, as a result of it becoming infected after the replacement operation. This restricts the information that my brain receives from my legs and I sway about very easily. I have taught myself to feel my feet and feel my knees, and to be careful how I move. I wear a built-up shoe and an elbow-crutch to support the side of me that has no joint.

In winter, or whenever it is slippery, I go very slowly on pavements, crawling along while I look down for treacherous glass lights and uneven paving stones. My progress is minute, but I respect my natural urge for caution.

One thing I do like is walking with one hand on a man's shoulder. Men are very much steadier, more solid, than women, I have found; holding on like that I feel safe, and can go more quickly than by myself.

## Exercise and Movement

A list of exercises can be very forbidding. People think, 'Do I have to do *all* that just to relieve a tiny bit of my pain?' So they don't do anything at all.

I hate the word 'exercise': 'movement' is a much better word for putting the idea over to people, because then you can explain what is going on. You move your hands to dress yourself, to put your bra on, to pull up your knickers, to eat your food – these movements are all part of a normal way of living. They are things that people want to go on being able to do.

So, if you are always dropping your food because your hands are weak, it makes sense to strengthen them so you do not drop your food. What is also certain is this: if you do nothing about it, it will only get worse.

It is a question of attitude. The more you let yourself be overtaken by your condition, the more I think you have to find out what you are here for. As a Scot, I was brought up to believe that life was service, that you automatically did things to help other people. Perhaps we carried that tradition too far, but the reverse is far more unacceptable. When people with arthritis huddle up in a corner and can only say, 'Oh, my poor back', they are electing out of life. I think you have to try and stay *in* life.

I recently interviewed a woman on television who had rheumatoid arthritis and osteoporosis (thinning of the bones). She had just been treated, marvellously, at Bath hospital, and I asked her to show me how she had sat before her treatment. She bent right forward, with her nose pointing down.

I said, 'How did you see through your glasses?'

'Oh,' she said, 'I couldn't see through them. I had to look over the top.'

Then she showed me how she sat now. Not only was she straight and able to use her glasses properly, she had also gained ½ in (1.25 cm) in height and 5 in (12.5 cm) in 'straightness'. This is a special measurement taken from the front of the ear to the wall behind: as she gradually straightened, this woman had pushed her head back 5 in (12.5 cm) closer to the wall.

I asked her what she had had to do to make such an improvement. She told me, and it seemed rather a lot, a good deal more than the two minutes an hour that I was used to. I asked her if it was worth it.

'Oh, certainly!' she said. Her face was smooth and happy. She looked like a going concern, not like a poor defeated thing. Later someone asked her why she had wanted to be on the programme.

'Because I want other people to realize that they don't have to stay as they are,' she said. 'It may not be possible for them to be cured, but they can be made to feel so much better. And their pain can go.'

Her outlook was so right. The stretching exercises had both straightened her *and* relieved the pressure on her spine. This in turn had taken away her pain. To put it another way: your head weighs about 12 lb (5.5 kg) and each arm about the same. If your body collapses forward past the straight-upright line, you will have the equivalent of nearly 3 st (19 kg) of potatoes pulling you forward. This puts enormous pressure on the spinal joints and on the nerves that come out between those joints; but if you can relieve that pressure, you relieve the pain.

Once people understand these principles, they are much more inclined to help themselves. Fortunately, the principles are not difficult to understand, and people are not daft. At heart, everyone wants to get better.

# Don't Overdo It

Pain is always a danger sign. It is there to stop you doing something. Once you have received the signal, look around to see what is causing it. You should never say, when exercising, 'Go through the burn.' When you feel this 'burn', or acute pain, it is because the lactic acid in your muscles is screaming out that you have abused your body. Listen to your pain, and try to find a more gentle solution.

# Hypothermia

People with arthritis who move slowly and are getting on in years face the additional danger of hypothermia. With advancing age, the inbuilt system for controlling body temperature grows less efficient. Elderly people lose heat without realizing it; they don't feel that they are cold – and that can be fatal.

If this state – of being cold but not aware of it – goes on for too long, you may suddenly start to feel strange, on the verge of fainting. You will gradually lose control of yourself, and will soon be unable to move your limbs. The reason for this is that your blood withdraws into your core – that is, the centre of you – to keep you alive, leaving you with less blood for your limbs and brain. This has happened to me on two occasions when I stayed out in the garden too long, and it is a problem that all people with arthritis should be wary of.

If you stay in this condition, you will die, eventually. The difficulty, when you feel this light-headedness coming on and cannot move your limbs properly, is to get yourself into the house and into warmth. There is no set procedure for dealing with this problem, but it is bound to help if you follow these guidelines:

1 Do not stay out in the cold too long.
2 Always wear several layers of warm clothing when you are outdoors and not moving much, as is often the case with gardeners.
3 As soon as you feel at all exhausted, get into the house *immediately.*

The procedure then is clear. Make the room warm if you can do so quickly, then get into bed and stay there. In that way you can conserve your own heat and re-establish control of your metabolism. Do not bother with hot-water bottles: you may burn yourself, and in any case your priority is to get into bed. If a friend is there, he or she can give you a warm drink, which you should take slowly. But remember: no hot drinks and no alcohol.

## Getting Up in the Night

If you usually have to get up at night to go to the lavatory, give careful thought to your predicament in advance. Do you have to totter about in the dark, or semi-dark, or go along cold passageways where you might slip, or climb up or down stairs?

You can make life much easier by having a commode beside the bed. I had one for quite some time when my legs were very bad. If you don't know where to get one, or you can't afford to buy one, ask the District Health Authority (DHA). They may be able to lend you one and empty it every day if you need this.

Everyone with arthritis should have a warm dressing gown, and warm slippers which the feet can slide into easily. These should be worn whenever he or she gets up in the night, for whatever reason.

Incidentally, the Victorians were right about nightcaps. We lose about one third of our body heat through our heads, and if you like an airy bedroom, as I do, a woolly hat is a good idea. Keep your extremities warm, too. Wear mittens or some kind of glove, if you like, and bedsocks. For sitting up in bed, or simply for covering your shoulders, a shawl is most helpful. Put it round across your front and tuck it in behind you. If you have not used a shawl before, you will find it a great comfort.

# AIDS AROUND THE HOME

Helpful items on display at the Disabled Living Foundation's Aids Centre in London include the following:

## Mobility

- Walking sticks; crutches; walking frames (ordinary, fold-up, with built-in seat, etc.); rollators (walking frames with two or four wheels)
- Wheelchairs, self-propelled or attendant-pushed; battery-driven power chairs, for indoor and outdoor use; 'runaround' scooters
- Shopping trolleys
- Stair lift

## Beds and chairs

- Beds and accessories; hoists for transferring from chair to bed, etc.
- High-seat chairs, some electrically or mechanically operated
- Blocks for raising height of beds and chairs

## Communications

- Environmental control systems (suck-blow switch for operating domestic appliances)
- Possum (POSM or Patient Operated Selected Mechanism), as supplied by DHSS on assessment, operating alarm, call phone, intercom, heater, television, radio, curtains, page turners, etc. (see also 'Life in a Wheelchair', page 38)
- Alarm systems

■ Telephone appliances – push-button controls;
stands for holding receiver

## General gadgets

■ Key turners; knob turners for doors; writing
aids; book rests; mechanized page turners;
'helping hands' or pick-up sticks
■ Gripkit, which moulds to a desired shape – for
example, for a key turner – and then hardens

## Clothing

■ Advice on dressing; dressing aids
■ Clothing and footwear

For further information, see the 'Help' section at the
end of the book and the chapter 'One Step Ahead'.

# IN THE KITCHEN

## Ann Macfarlane

Ann Macfarlane writes on cookery for *Arthritis News* and has recently published a book, *Are You Cooking Comfortably?* She contracted Still's Disease (juvenile chronic arthritis) at the age of four and spent long periods living at home, in hospital or in a residential home until, in 1974, she went to live on her own in a flat in Surbiton, Surrey. Here she discusses the problems and satisfactions of independent eating and cooking.

Diet is a subject for the experts and at the moment there is not a lot they agree about! It is an important subject for people with arthritis because many are seeking answers about which foods may suit them best. Unfortunately, I fear we shall have to wait some time yet before firm advice can be given.

In the meantime, and before we go into the kitchen, I will pass quickly to a related subject that interests many of us – our weight and how much food we should eat. Many people with arthritis find that if they eat a normal amount of food, they put on weight. The reason for this is usually because they are so immobile; their bodies have no chance to burn off the surplus energy and therefore it is converted to fat. This is by no means true of everyone. Some people may find a normal diet inadequate for their needs and actually lose weight. For others, it is more important to find a correct balance between what they eat and the drugs they have to take. These are all medical problems and should therefore be discussed with a doctor.

People with arthritis who do have a weight problem, or whose family history leads them to think that they will have a weight problem if they go on eating and being immobile at their current rates, really should try to do something about it.

This is not easy, I know. People with a lot of time to fill, or who are not feeling well, or who can't get motivated, often turn to food as a form of comfort or entertainment. In my own case, I had to do something drastic about my weight. In my late teens and early twenties I was obese-plus-plus: over 16 st (100 kg) and only 5 ft (1.5 m) tall. Unhappy with the negative advice I had been receiving from doctors, I then did a very silly thing: I put myself on a crash diet. I lost weight all right, but it did not do my health any good. Fortunately, I then found a sympathetic doctor and became more sensible.

Nowadays (that was all a few years ago!) there are more opportunities for getting personal advice about your diet. As well as your doctor there are community nutritionists who can be visited, and it should not be difficult to sort out a balanced diet appropriate to your weight and general health.

Right. That's enough about the theory of eating. Let's now go into ...

## The Impossible Room

Designing a perfect kitchen for someone with arthritis is almost an impossible task. The main requirement is that, ideally, everything should be on the same level, but this can be a problem. Out would go all those high cupboards you can't reach into; out would go all those low cupboards that are just as awkward and painful to use. Instead, your sinks, work surfaces and storage units would extend in a huge kind of ribbon development – but that would be no good, either, because you would need an enormous room to contain everything; and you wouldn't like that because of all the fetching and carrying.

The answer, as usual, is a compromise, and this is where you can and should seek help. If your kitchen does not work for you, or your arthritis is causing you new problems, or you are newly disabled, ask an occupational therapist to come and advise. Kitchen planning is one of their fields of expertise, and they may recommend anything from a minor rearrangement of your shelves to a much more radical alteration for which builders would be needed. If finance is a problem, don't forget that you may be able to obtain a grant for this work: the *Disability Rights Handbook* (see page 150) gives useful advice on this subject.

My flat is in a block that was purpose-built about ten years ago for disabled people. Design for the disabled was then in its early stages, and my kitchen rather reflects this. It compares reasonably well with some of the latest designs which I have seen, but it does have its drawbacks.

For instance, I have a beautiful built-in oven which I never use. When I am in the kitchen, I am in a wheelchair with my legs extended. This makes for quite a few difficulties, one of which is that the oven is completely out of my reach. (I use a multi-cooker instead.) I also find that the sink is painful to use because it is too deep; a shallower one would be better for me because I would not have to reach so far into it. The fridge, too, is awkwardly positioned in a corner; I have to open the door with a special gadget and use a 'helping hand' to lift things in and out.

I am planning to have some alterations made to my kitchen which will make life easier. In the meantime, I have learnt to adapt to these difficulties, partly with the help of certain gadgets and partly by thinking out my problems very carefully. For example, I have half a dozen 'helping hands' around my flat, and they can do a lot of tasks for me. I also have a special gadget which is invaluable. It consists of a stick with a cup hook screwed into one end and a thimble over the other end. My brother-in-law makes them for me. I use the hook for opening doors, for lifting cups by the handle and all sorts of other things. If I drop something on the floor – which I often do – I can sometimes pick it up by pushing the thimble end of the stick inside the object and levering it into the air. If that doesn't work I always have plenty of plastic bags available; I then push the object inside the bag and use my stick to lift the bag. It took me ages to figure this out, but now it saves me a lot of time and spares me a great deal of frustration.

Today there are all kinds of kitchen aids on the market. By far the best place to view them is the Aids Centre of the Disabled Living Foundation (see page 33). Your occupational therapist will also be able to advise you about particular kitchen items; if you have not tried to cook for yourself before, it is a big help to have someone show you what is available and how to use it.

My main piece of advice about kitchen equipment is this: think before you buy. You can waste an awful lot of money if you don't quite know what you are looking for. One way to establish what you need is to plan a weekly menu and then see what kind of equipment you will have to buy to produce all those dishes. If the list is too big, you can always modify the menu!

For me the first essential is a good sharp knife. If you have not discovered this already, you will be surprised just how much you can achieve with one good knife. Then you will need to look at all the devices for preparing food, cooking it and serving it. Some disabled people find a food processor invaluable. Personally I do not want one because there are too many bits and attachments to assemble and clean. I prefer to keep things as simple as possible.

For tasks such as peeling vegetables, or holding something steady, like a kettle, there are various gadgets available. Try to see as many different ones as you can before you buy. What kind of pots and pans you choose will depend on the type of cooking you plan to do. In general, I recommend lightweight pans, bowls and dishes – to make lifting easier – and non-stick surfaces to save time and labour when it comes to washing up.

Think also about how you want to drain food. There are various ways to avoid lifting heavy, water-filled pans; for instance, by ladling the contents out, or having a frying basket inside the pan which you lift out, disposing of the water later.

Always consider your disability before you buy anything, whether it be a cooking utensil or something on your regular shopping list. I would never buy a large, economy-size bottle of washing-up liquid, for example; the bottle is too big for me to get my hands round. I could, of course, still save some money by buying it and then dispensing the liquid into smaller containers, but this is a lot of hassle and I have decided against doing it. Incidentally, I find waisted bottles are better for me; these are slowly coming into the shops and I welcome them.

I use very few cans – they are heavy to carry home and heavy to lift in and out of cupboards – but if I do buy them I usually get a small size. Then there is a the problem of opening them. I have a special can-opener which I am able to operate. If the contents of the can are solid, I don't mind opening it myself; if they are liquid (either entirely or partly, as with canned fruit in juice), then I may ask someone else to do it for me. The labour of clearing up the spillage is something I can do without.

For similar reasons I don't buy food in bulk to store in the freezer. It may save money to do so but I prefer not to have the bother of loading and unloading, defrosting and so on. I know from experience that it is not cost-effective for my temper or for my physical wellbeing. I proved this to myself a long time ago. When I was first trying to be independent, I bought a small chicken for my supper. I cooked it and took it out of the oven, then the dish slipped in my hand and it all ended up on the floor. It took me three hours to clean up the mess. I was exhausted. I learned there and then to live within my abilities. Modern techniques of food preparation have made it unnecessary for me to spend hours trying to cook something and bring it successfully to the table. I know there is a world of difference in taste between an oven-ready slice of meat and gravy and a joint that I have cooked myself. However, I find it better to take the easy option and eliminate the possibility of all that agony and frustration when it goes wrong.

## Who Will Do the Shopping?

It makes better sense if whoever is doing the cooking also does the shopping. Cooks know their budget best, which brands they like, and can plan more effectively if they actually go out and buy their ingredients. For some people, however, this is impossible – they are too disabled – in which case the job has to be done by someone else. Others, although they may be able to get to the shops, don't feel well enough – perhaps they are suffering from fatigue and decide they must cut down on their general workload – so their shopping is delegated.

There is also the person who can still cope, but who wishes that shopping was not such a hassle. Here are some ideas for making shopping trips less troublesome.

Ask your supermarket when the shop is least crowded, then time your visits to fit those hours. It really does make a difference.

Don't be afraid to ask for help. Get a friend to go with you, who can pick things off the shelves for you, load and unload the trolley; or, if you go alone, ask if one of the assistants can help you. This is what I now do and it works perfectly well. It took me several years to suppress my pride, mind you, but once I had asked I found that the shop assistants were only too pleased and willing to help. Now I get around the supermarket in ten to fifteen minutes instead of fifty.

I also have a money problem when I go shopping: I can't grip coins properly and they constantly end up on the floor. The solution? Pay by cheque. Pre-write it so you only have to insert the amount and sign it.

# KITCHEN AIDS

Helpful items on display at the Disabled Living Foundation's Aids Centre in London include the following:

## Kitchen units and cookers

- Units fixed at wheelchair height, with extra pull-out working surfaces; corner cupboard with automatic lifting bin and carousel (swing-out) storage trays
- Sink unit, adjustable height
- Split-level cooker

## Gadgets

- Jar openers; belly clamp to hold jar in place; can openers; tap turner; kettle and teapot tippers; drinking vessels – mugs and cups; assorted cutlery; trays for carrying one-handed; buttering boards; long-handled dustpans and brushes; umbrella-handled milk bottle holder
- Trolleys for carrying food, which also provide a walking aid
- Perching stool

## *In Touch* kitchen

- A fully fitted kitchen designed for the partially sighted and organized in collaboration with the *In Touch* BBC radio programme.

## Gas and electricity

- Controls for cookers, plugs and other appliances, organized in collaboration with the gas and electricity authorities' Home Adviser schemes.

---

For further information, see the 'Help' section at the end of the book and the chapter 'One Step Ahead'.

# IN THE
# BATHROOM

Bathroom design has greatly improved in recent years and there are now aids and gadgets to suit almost every need and preference. They range from such wonders as the bath with hydraulic base, which rises up to receive the bather transferring from a wheelchair and then lowers him or her gently into the water, to toothbrushes with built-up handles which are easier to grip.

Showers are becoming increasingly popular among those who find it a struggle to get in and out of a bath. For others, who do not have this problem, it seems as though nothing can compare with a lovely restful soak in warm water.

Some bathroom aids are expensive and people may be deterred by this from trying to obtain one that would really help them. If this applies to you, don't forget that you may be able to get a special bath or other aid through the Social Services. They employ community occupational therapists, or rehabilitation officers as some are called, who visit people at home to assess their need for aids and adaptations. If the aid is portable, they provide it on an indefinite loan basis. If it is fixed – a bath, say, or even a complete new bathroom or kitchen installation – then a grant can be made available which is usually for 75 per cent of the total cost. The grant may be higher, subject to a means test, and it also varies according to which Social Services area the applicant lives in. For further information, see the 'Help' section at the end of the book.

The next two contributions consider practical aspects relating to the bathroom. As they clearly show, choosing, or making, equipment for the bathroom is very much a matter for the individual.

# A SHOWER FOR ME

## Phil Smith

Phil Smith, who later describes how she copes as a mum with arthritis (see page 70), here talks about her bathroom.

I now have a walk-in shower, and am very glad that I do. It is something that I evolved towards over the years as I came to realize that a bath was not the best solution for someone with my kind of rheumatoid arthritis.

When we had only a bath, I had to wait until my husband was at home so he could put me into it. He would then leave me there and go downstairs. I used to think, 'It's been a long day, so I'll have a nice soak.'

Time went by. The water grew cold, but I could not turn on the tap to run some more hot water. By then I would be getting distinctly cold, so I would call to Rich to come and get me out; but, because I didn't want to wake the kids, I would try to call out quietly. And, of course, quite often he didn't hear me. He'd be downstairs thinking, 'She's having a lovely long soak tonight,' when all I wanted was to escape from the thing.

With the shower everything is much easier. I walk straight into it and have none of the bother of climbing in or out as I did with the bath. The on/off tap is larger, too, with indentations round the side which make it easier to grip, and in addition I have a lever attached to mine so that I can work the tap with a simple turning movement.

I also have a raised toilet seat, which is so much easier. I'd had arthritis for nine years before I got one, mainly because, early on, nobody told me about them, but also, partly, because of pride. I used to tell myself that I could manage. In fact, it makes such a difference, helping you to cope on your own instead of having to rely on others, that I now recommend them to anyone who has difficulty in lowering themselves on to a seat and raising themselves up again.

# POKER STICKS AND
# THROWTHROUGHS

## Alice Pearl

Alice Pearl, who maintains her independent spirit despite being bedbound, here describes her solution to an awkward problem.

The only parts of me that I am able to wash are my hands, face and bottom; and I could not wash *that* part of me without one of the special pokers that I make for myself.

This is one aspect of being disabled which can be very hard to bear. You can't hide it; it has got to be faced. Nature has its way and you must cope with that from one day to the next.

With my arthritis I had got to a stage where I could not keep myself clean, and I was worried to death about it. So I made these pokers and they do the trick.

A poker consists of a wooden stick with a piece of foam secured over one end with elastic bands.* I make sure I have several available all the time. When used with the special soap provided for me by my doctor (because I have had skin trouble in the past) I can give myself a good wash. Afterwards I dry myself by throwing a towel through my legs with one hand and catching it on the other side with the other; then I see-saw with the towel, backwards and forwards, until I am dry.

When the nurses come, they wash my body for me in the shower. My routine with the pokers, however, enables me to keep myself clean in between times.

*Editor's Note:* Ready-made bottom washers can now be bought – see 'Bathroom Aids' panel (opposite).

# BATHROOM AIDS

Helpful items on display at the Disabled Living Foundation's Aids Centre in London include the following:

## Washing equipment

■ Long-handled brushes for reaching toes; bottom washers; nail brushes mounted on two suction cups; two-handled towelling strip for reaching the back; toothbrushes with built-up handles for easier grip

## Baths, basins and showers

■ Many types of bath to suit individual needs – for example, with side door for easier access and a tipping device which allows water to flow over occupant (de luxe model and expensive, but remember that grants are available on assessment from the Social Services)

■ Bath boards and seats which can be built into the bath itself; non-slip mats for use in bath; hoists to help access

■ Showers with or without seats; non-slip mats

■ Lever taps – easier to turn than crystal or criss-cross types

## Toilets and bidets

■ Raised toilet seats for fitting to standard toilets; toilet frame; bidets; commodes

■ Grab rails to help with getting up and down – for use anywhere in the bathroom

For further information, see the 'Help' section at the end of the book.

# LIFE IN A WHEELCHAIR

## Pamela La Fane

Pamela La Fane spends all her days in a wheelchair. She first began to suffer from rheumatoid arthritis (Still's Disease) at the age of eleven while she was a wartime evacuee in Oxfordshire. In a very short time she could do almost nothing for herself, and when she was sixteen she was sent back to London and put into a geriatric hospital. There she was told, 'We don't give any treatment ... no-one gets better here.' In her book, *It's A Lovely Day, Outside*, she has written movingly of how she fought her disability and prison-like surroundings until, in 1968, she was allowed to leave and live in a specially fitted ground-floor council flat in South London.

I have been living in my flat for eighteen years. To begin with, I had an unmarried mother to live in and help me. When she left to get married I carried on this arrangement with other girls who had babies and needed a home to bring them up in, either until they got married or went off to do something else with their lives. For the most part I got on fine with a lot of the girls and one delightful Australian girl stayed with me for two and a half years. Some of the others, however, had problems: one, it turned out, was on probation for stealing, but at the time we didn't know that – not until we found that she'd been helping herself to my bank balance!

After that, the Social Services and I agreed that we'd better find another sort of scheme, so now I have two ladies who live here, one week on and one week off. They are both middle-aged with grown-up families, and they are much more practical and reliable. One of them, Betty, has been here nine and a half years.

My physical condition now is much the same as it was when I came here, and I don't expect it to change. My joints are all ankylosed (rigid) and this is the way they will stay. I have had occasional flare-ups but normally I don't receive treatment and

I don't take any drugs, except perhaps aspirin to relieve pain on the odd occasion.

My power-drive chair is everything to me. It has taken over the job my legs once did for me, but have not been able to do since I was a child. If ever it breaks down I get very bad-tempered because it means waiting several days while it is repaired, and instead I have to use my ordinary wheelchair, which doesn't give me any mobility unless someone pushes it.

Using the power chair, I can drive myself round the flat, which has specially widened doors and a ramp to enable me to get out through the back door. The only other alteration the builders had to make in my flat was to the bathroom. I couldn't turn my chair and get in through the ordinary door from the hall, so they made me another entrance direct from my bedroom. Otherwise, my flat is the same as the others in the block.

## The Possum and Me

To help me do things when I am on my own I have a Possum unit – Possum stands for 'Patient Operated Selected Mechanism'. It has an indicator board with switches that operate the front door, turn on the light and the television, and perform a variety of other functions. Mine is one of the earliest Possums, less sophisticated than later models, but it still works, and that's the important thing.

Because my fingers are too rigid for me to be able to press switches, I use a special stick, which I push between my fingers. At the top of the Possum's indicator board there is a lit switch marked 'START'. To call up one of the operations I hold down this master switch with my stick while a light moves round the board. When it reaches the operation I want I push the switch to hold it, and then that particular operation is automatically carried out.

There are six main switches on my Possum, as follows:

'SOS'. In theory, when this goes off, everyone comes rushing to help. I came back once after a day out and found that one of my cats had sat on the switch and activated the SOS. Goodness knows how many hours it had been ringing, but nobody had come. However, if I *was* alone in dire trouble, I would put the SOS on *and* the intercom, so it could be heard outside the front door; otherwise it doesn't carry far enough.

'AID'. I use this buzzer to call one of the ladies in the flat if she hasn't heard me. I can also use it if I want something during the night, because it's wired through to the bedroom and I can operate it from my bed.

'INTERCOM'. This is connected to the entry phone in the hall of my flat. I can't go out and pick up the entry phone like an able-bodied person so this enables me to let visitors in through the outer door and then speak to them on the intercom when they reach my front door. Then I operate...

'DOOR'. This lets them into the flat. It's all very high-tech, as you can see!

'LIGHT'. This puts on the side light in my main room.

'HEAT'. In the winter I can use this to turn on an electric fire. I don't often need this because the flat is centrally heated, but if the heating ever goes wrong I have got this as a back-up.

In addition, I can switch on my television with the Possum, using a remote-controlled handset to select the channels, adjust the picture and so on. There are also two other signs on the indicator board – 'RADIO' and 'INTERNAL BELL' – but I don't need these because I have a transistor radio I can work myself, and the 'AID' buzzer does the work of the internal bell.

As well as the Possum I also have a special phone. Because I can't get my arms up, this phone is adapted so that I can simply work one switch to get a dialling tone and then another one, called a 'sender', to reach the operator on Special Service. She knows I am a disabled caller and will get the number for me.

These three pieces of equipment – the power chair, the Possum unit and the special phone – are extremely important to me. Without them I would not have any degree of mobility or independent life.

## Writing – A Way Out

I also rely very much on my lady helpers. One of them has to be there first thing in the morning to help me get up, and to wash and dress me. At night there is the reverse process, so that I can be put to bed. In between, whoever is living in does all the shopping and cooking, the washing, ironing and housework.

About the only physical thing I can do completely on my own is write. I fit the pen, an ordinary biro, between my thumb and forefinger and off I go. I have an electronic typewriter as well, which I can work with my special stick.

Thanks to writing, I now have my own transport – a Ford Transit van which I bought with the proceeds from my first book. I can't drive it myself, of course, and neither of my two ladies can drive, so it's a problem finding a driver. I know two chaps who are very good, but they both work full-time and are only free at the weekends. Sometimes it can be very frustrating, wanting to go out and knowing the van is just sitting there.

On the other hand, I am very glad I've got it. It has meant that I have been able to spread my wings and travel to places I would never have seen otherwise. I have been to the Continent, visited Paris and Brussels – things I could not have dreamt of doing all those years I was shut away in hospital.

Before I came to this flat, travelling for pleasure had always been completely out of the question. Then, after I had settled in here, I began to wonder. I was very happy to have joined the 'outside world'; now I wanted to see more of it. I was not totally confined to my four walls because the girls could push me around the local streets in a wheelchair, but I never really got beyond Wandsworth or Putney. Having the vehicle has made a world of difference.

People ask me what I do with myself all day. They see me in the wheelchair and think I must get bored easily, but in fact I find the time goes quickly. I try to do some writing every day, and am working on another book at the moment. I belong to a local writers' group and I have a lot of other interests, too, so passing the time is not a problem. My life is stable. The arthritis is dormant most of the time, and I have learned to adapt to my disabilities and to do everything in the way that I find easiest.

Sometimes a neighbour may say something to Betty like, 'Oh, that poor woman, that poor woman.' Betty tells them, 'You don't have to say that about Pam. She lives a perfectly normal life.' I suppose it must be difficult for some people with arthritis, particularly if they are in pain all the time, but I like to think that I *do* lead a normal life. The only difference is that I am not mobile.

If I were allowed one special wish, I would ask for a permanent full-time chauffeur [*laughter*]. Apart from that I am quite satisfied.

# FOR THE
# BEDBOUND

## Alice Pearl

Alice Pearl is virtually confined to bed. She developed rheumatoid arthritis at the age of eighteen, and at first was able to adapt to it: she married, had a child and looked after the family home. Now a widow, she has struggled to cope with the encroachments of the disease even though they have left her severely disabled, with both knees and hips fused. She lives, as independently as she can, with her dog and cat in a bungalow in Nottingham, and until recently was transport officer for her local branch of Arthritis Care.

Disabled as I am, there are still a lot of things I can manage for myself. I can no longer walk in the garden as I used to, and I must watch my diet carefully. One of the things that happens when you are immobile is that you tend to put on weight, and that's no use. I have a hiatus hernia on top of all the arthritis and so I have to keep to a fat-free diet. One must eat – but reasonably.

I have been in this bungalow since 1970. Before that we lived in a big house with lots of stairs. I still think of it as home, but I couldn't cope there because of my disability so we came here. Then, after a very serious illness, my husband died. I tried to struggle on by myself but I could never get done with the housework. I decided to move into one room and reorganize the way I live.

In this room I have an electric bed which tilts forward to put me in an upright position, and from there I can get hold of my trolley and push myself to the bathroom and the kitchen, and back again. It takes a long time but I can do it. When I first got this bed it didn't have a motor, just a handle which I couldn't turn. After six months it was fitted with a motor from Germany and it has been good for me ever since. Nurses come in the morning to wash and dress me, and put on my long-leg splints and boots, and in the evening they come and take everything off so I can settle for the night. Otherwise, I manage by myself. I am very well organized, as I have to be, and keep the things I need around me, at the ready.

I have had my setbacks, and at one time I was very ill – I think from a drug that went wrong on me – and never left my bed for five weeks. They had to get night nurses in for me. I began to think I would be stuck there for the rest of my life, so one day I asked the nurse to put my boots on for me.

'Whatever for?' she asked.

'Please will you put on my boots,' I insisted.

She did as I asked, and tilted the bed so that my feet were on the floor. I got hold of my trolley and stood there for a while until it ached too much and I had to go back to bed.

The next day I took two or three steps, leaning on my trolley. Another day I got as far as the sideboard. One Sunday, I actually got myself into the kitchen. I was so pleased, I rang my daughter: 'Betty,' I cried, 'I've got into the kitchen!'

Gradually I got back so I was all right and could do things again. My brain still ticks over, and if I wasn't so immobile I would do a lot more.

## Daily Duties

In its normal horizontal position my bed is quite high off the ground – about 2 ft 6 in (0.75 m). This means I am raised up almost to the level of my window and have a lovely view out to the garden. On shelves or stands on either side of the bed I keep supplies of everything I will need, all within easy reach. These include my stores of tea, dried milk, sugar in small containers, and my tablets and creams. There is a panel of power points – one for the bed, one for the television, one for the kettle, and so on. I also have my telephone, a light, a drawer for my personal things and papers, and a pull-out tray which I put my meals on. It may look like a lot of untidy clutter, but in fact it is all part of my special system; and it works.

I start the day at six o'clock with my first cup of tea, which I put honey in. I do my scripture reading and say my prayers. I wash my hands, using a cloth wetted with surgical spirit, and then I am ready for my breakfast, which I prepare the day before and bring through after tea. After that the nurses arrive to wash and dress me.

My trolley is very important to me. When the bed tilts forward, I grasp my stick, which is hanging nearby, and push myself into a standing position on a slip mat. I reach forward for the rail on the trolley, which looks like a tea trolley and was specially made for me, and then I can push myself through to the kitchen. I keep a portable telephone on the trolley so that I can call for help if I end up on the floor. That has happened several times – I can never be sure I will keep my balance!

Once I've got to the kitchen, where everything is kept on one level because I can't bend down or reach up, I prop myself against the units on my elbows and drag myself across to the microwave. This has been invaluable to me. I can boil milk in it, bake potatoes for myself, and cook the meat for the dog and the cat, which I feed myself. I stay in the kitchen for about an hour, then I push back to my bed. I rest until dinner, which is brought by Meals-on-Wheels, and then I rest again. At about two o'clock I push through to the kitchen and get my tea ready. Sometimes my home help gets a salad ready for me, and sometimes I make it myself. I take this back to bed on the trolley, and then at five o'clock I push through again to have a wash and clear up the tea things. The nurses come back between six o'clock and eight o'clock to take my splints off and put me to bed, where I stay till morning.

During the day I keep myself on the go like that because I know it helps me. Just lying in bed all the time is no good for the circulation, and it makes you sore as well.

A home help comes in for two hours, five mornings a week. On Sundays I have what we call a 'pop-in', but that leaves me on Saturdays with nobody, although the nurses come in every day.

I decided early on that if I was going to spend my life in one room I would make it as interesting as possible to look at. I could not bear to have tidy blank walls. My favourite colour is red and I've got all sorts of red things in the room, as well as pictures and little treasures which people bring me.

I always have plenty to do. I like to keep up with current affairs on the radio; I do a lot of crosswords; and I also organize the entertainment for my branch of Arthritis Care. People pop in throughout the day, whether it's the nurses or the home help, the dinner lady or the library lady, or the priest who brings me Holy Communion. I have had as many as ten people in here at the same time – not because I was giving a party, but because they had just turned up together.

## Learning from Nature

As I've said, through the window I have a lovely view into the garden. I can push open the window to feed the birds, and someone fills the birdbath for me so that I get plenty of visitors. I have a name for all the birds which come, and I get great satisfaction from watching them.

I believe we have a lot to learn from Nature. Especially when I am in pain and it is a struggle to get started in the morning, I look out there at the trees and the birds and take comfort. I remind myself that in the garden there is one beautiful tree – and another that is not so beautiful. Yet they both function; they both have a purpose.

Then along comes a poor little pigeon with only one claw. He still gets on with his life, despite the limitations he must put up with. He gets his food and seems happy enough, so far as I can tell. That, to me, is normal. Just because some of us are disabled, there is no need to be depressed and miserable about it.

Why should we all expect to be standard?

# WHEN WILL THEY DO IT BETTER?

## Jo Richardson

Design for the disabled has made great advances in the last few years. What often lags behind is human understanding on the part of architects, builders, and the army of skilled tradesmen and engineers who fit things in our homes. Jo Richardson, MP, who talks about her rheumatoid arthritis later in the book (see page 106), here describes some of the domestic horrors she has come across. Readers who have also suffered – you are not alone!

Since the beginning of the seventies it has gradually become accepted that the disabled should have special facilities. I can now go to a political meeting and find the organizers apologizing if they haven't managed to book a hall which has those facilities. Before it would not have entered their heads to ask for them.

However, the actual provision of facilities is not nearly what it should be. The majority of public buildings are not set up for disabled people. In future we ought to write into the design of every new building a requirement that proper thought must be given to disabled users. This would apply to private houses, flats, shops, offices, factories, public buildings – everywhere a disabled person is likely to go. In the meantime, I come across some dreadful instances of disabled people being messed about by housing authorities, builders, and people who should know a great deal better.

In one case a daughter, aged forty-five and severely disabled, lived with her mother, aged seventy-eight. The daughter could only get out of her wheelchair to roll onto her bed. After three years of battling with the local bureaucracy it was agreed they could have a shower because the mother was no longer able to lift her quite heavy daughter in and out of the bath.

The bathroom was redesigned. When the mother saw the plans she immediately realized that they would not work. The basin, the shower and the toilet had each been pushed into a corner. She explained that her daughter would not be able to get up to the basin because the arms of her wheelchair would hit the walls.

'No, dear,' said the authorities. 'You're wrong.'

They ignored her and the conversion work began. As it went on, the mother grew increasingly worried that she would not be able to wash her daughter if the shower was placed in a corner of the room. It would only be open on two sides and she needed three to get round the other side of the wheelchair.

'No, dear,' said the authorities. 'This is the most suitable place. We know best.'

They took all the old fittings out – toilet, bath, the lot – and left the mother and daughter with nothing for seven weeks. Then they put the new basin in one corner and the shower in another corner.

This appalling saga went on for several more episodes until, finally, the new basin in the corner was ripped out and a bigger, more suitable one installed against one wall, and the shower moved to where it should have been all along.

If the mother and daughter had not remained astonishingly even-tempered throughout, I don't know what would have happened to them. In their place I would have gone barmy. As it was, the mother simply said to me, 'I don't know why it is, but I seem to cry more often these days.'

# Wanted: More Women in Charge

I honestly believe that everyone would benefit if there were more women planners, architects and designers. Historically, women have used the homes we live in more than men. This has given them a certain expertise in the way rooms should be designed and fitted out. Unfortunately, many women are too tied to their home and family to take on the extra commitment that this requires.

It is true that some women are coming through the relevant professions, but only in very small numbers. If you go into any local authority planning department you will see women doing tracing work; but the people on the drawing boards – actually doing the designs – are men. I think we miss something through this. Women could contribute so much that would be good and useful, but they will not be able to do so until they are somehow relieved of their domestic obligations. In the meantime, I wish that those who make the decisions would listen more carefully to women; even ask their advice.

I had another case recently where the local authority had put in a new bathroom. To do so, they had extended the building at the back and, by cutting new doorways, had fixed it so that access to all the rooms at the back was from one tiny hallway onto which all the doors opened inwards. It was ludicrous. I said so to the borough architect.

'How do people manage?' I asked him.

'Perfectly OK,' he said. 'We do this often. You just have to make sure nobody's coming through one of the other doors at the same time as you.'

The woman who lived there, and who complained to me, had seen what was wrong from the beginning. The architect, on the other hand, couldn't see a problem even after it was built. That's what I mean about a woman's perspective having its uses.

## A Few Home Truths

I have a very nice flat. With a little more forethought it could have been even better. Here are just a few examples of the problems.

The kitchen is much too small – as all kitchens are. The top cupboards are so far out of reach, I would need to be 6 ft 4 in (1.95 m) to get the doors open, let alone put my hands inside. I have to stand on a stool to use them, which is not good for me because I don't have good balance; but it's daft anyway, for anyone. If the architects know the storage space is inadequate, why don't they make kitchens bigger?

Another thing. Why do all the power points have to be down by the skirting board? Why can't they be at hip level so I can use them more easily? It may have been more convenient for the chap who installed the wiring to run short spurs up through the floorboards, but it's not convenient for me – and I live there!

I have a phone that I plug into wall sockets. These too are down at floor level. The engineer brought me a new phone about a year ago and said he would have to change the fitment on the wall as well. I asked him if he would put the new one higher up the wall so it would be easier to reach.

'No,' he said, 'I don't think I can. I'll try, but I don't think I can.'

When he'd finished, he told me he *had* moved it up after all. I looked. It was true. He'd moved it up an inch (2.5 cm).

The electricity board sent me a card to say they had to come and do something to the meter. I fixed a time for them to come and a place for them to collect the keys. The meter is high up on the wall and I left them a note asking them to move it down so I could read it more easily when I filled in their cards.

I came back that evening. They had moved the meter up, not down, so it was almost scraping the ceiling. The dial was now impossible to read.

Perhaps if we all complained more often...?

# ONE STEP AHEAD

## Margaret Dowden

When Margaret Dowden knew she was going to have her hips replaced, she realized that life at home would not be the same after she came out of hospital. With the help of her friends at the Disabled Living Foundation, where she works, she planned a path for herself through the difficult months ahead.

Once I had a date for going into hospital, I began to think very carefully about what it would be like. From my friends at the DLF (Disabled Living Foundation) and my own experience of working with the disabled, I knew I would be very uncomfortable for quite a long time afterwards. However, I did not want to go into a convalescent home; I wanted to go back to my flat, where I lived alone. What should I do about it?

The main limiting factor would be bending down. If I could not bend down, there would be many things I would not be able to reach: plugs, for instance. Rather than have a lot of plaster ripped out so the power points could be raised, I went out and bought three extension leads. Each consisted of a length of cable with a plug on one end and a socket on the other. I placed the socket ends at convenient heights around my flat so that, for instance, I could plug in and unplug the television without having to bend.

A raised toilet seat would be essential, I knew (and so it proved). High-seat chairs, too, or at least a chair with a seat at a decent height. For someone like me, a dining chair is much better for relaxing in than a low armchair. People who come home from hospital and immediately flop into their favourite easy chair actually risk injuring themselves when they try to get out of it.

I did heaps of basic shopping in advance, so that I would not have to pester people all the time to get me this or that. I got extra coffee, extra tea, toilet paper, washing-up liquid, and so on; if it was bulky or fairly heavy, and durable as well, I bought it. I stocked up the store cupboard with tins and filled the deep freeze.

I also had to think about going *into* hospital. Was I prepared for that? The hospital provided nothing in the way of a list of what to bring. On my own initiative I bought a supply of shortie nighties, reasoning that there was little point in wearing voluminous full-length nightdresses if I was having a hip operation; also, hospitals are notoriously overheated.

The operation was successful. I survived the heat and came home. Shortly before I left hospital I was given a brief set of dos and don'ts, mainly aimed at ensuring that I did not promptly dislocate my new hip. No-one mentioned, however, that I would not be able to get in and out of the bath by myself. Fortunately, one of the girls from work brought me a bath board so that I could sit over the bath and swing my legs across. If you get one, by the way, make sure that the board is balanced firmly and does not slide about.

I did arrive home with one very useful implement which the hospital had given me. This was a long-handled shoehorn, which was very convenient for easing feet into shoes. It also had a hook on the other end and this was intended as an aid for pulling on knickers. If you have never thought about this before, there is no way of doing it by yourself without either bending (forbidden) or using some kind of aid to hoist them into place from a starting point somewhere around your ankles.

Other problems I had to solve by my own ingenuity. This could be both amusing and satisfying. One of my great joys of the day is my early-morning tea. However, once I was walking on elbow-crutches it was impossible to carry a cup of tea out of the kitchen. The solution, I discovered, was to take an ordinary tray with two handles and thread my dressing-gown cord through the handles to make a self-supporting tray like the old matchsellers carry. It worked better, admittedly, when I was able to have one hand free to steady the tray (as I grew stronger and discarded one crutch), but the great thing was that I had thought it out for myself, and that was very pleasing.

Sleeping, I have to say, was difficult. If you do not naturally sleep on your back, and I do not, then you have problems. Before I left hospital I was told that I must not lie on my non-operated side for six to eight weeks. This was because I might put out the new joint as I turned that leg over. I could lie on the operated side when I felt I could bear to, but of course I didn't want to for quite some while. I came out of the operating theatre with a pillow between my legs to stop me turning, and when I got home I carried on doing this as a reminder.

When I found I could sleep only intermittently, I tried to be positive about it. All right, I didn't sleep well; but I *was* back in my flat, where I most wanted to be. So, instead of lying there muttering and moaning that I could not sleep, I got up and made myself a cup of tea. In fact, this also did me good physically, because as I paced up and down the flat in the early hours, I was exercising the new joint – and exercise is what you must do.

People had warned me that I would find the physiotherapists a pretty rough lot. So they were, but I think they have to be. Perhaps some of their patients do not take them seriously enough, and so they set high exercise targets in the hope that the patient will at least do a reasonable amount if not all. Personally I am convinced that the exercises must be done. After a hip operation a lot of deep muscle has been quite seriously interfered with, and only by exercise can the patient get back to fitness.

To summarize: plan your life-after-hospital before you go in; move sensibly at all times, and avoid bending and low chairs; and do what your physiotherapist tells you to do. Oh, and don't be frightened of the operation. Compared with some of the things the surgeons can do nowadays, it is a very straightforward piece of work. After it's done and settled down, you should feel so much better; as I do.

# FURTHER WAYS TO
# ADAPT YOUR HOME

### Letter box

Fit a basket beneath your letter box to catch the
post and newspapers.

### Floor covering

Avoid loose rugs, carpets and mats. Holes in carpets
and lino are also dangerous, and so are trailing
wires.

### Hand rails

Fit these where you need extra support, perhaps on
both sides of the stairs or to help you up and down
the steps to the garden.

### Waste bins

Use a truck or trolley to ferry waste bins to the
main dustbin. Ask the dustmen to collect your bin(s)
from a point convenient to you.

### Bedding

Continental quilts are easier to manage than
blankets. If you prefer blankets, choose a
lightweight cellular type.

See also the other lists on pages 26, 33 and 37, and
refer to the 'Help' section at the end of the book.

# OUT AND ABOUT

## INTRODUCTION

In this section of the book we are concerned mainly with how people with arthritis manage when they have to go beyond their own front doors – on a shopping trip, to work, to visit friends and relatives, or for any one of a hundred other reasons that are their business entirely.

## Public Transport

Public transport is undoubtedly the bugbear. So many of the contributors we spoke to have given it up altogether, or use it so sparingly, that if they are typical of other arthritis sufferers it begins to look as though public transport is not really public at all, but a series of services reserved for agile individuals.

### Buses

People were rudest about buses. It certainly seems time for a big rethink about buses and what they are for. The present design concept is much the same as it was when they were drawn by horses: a lurching passenger box, on one or two levels, with dauntingly steep winding stairs and aisles impassable to anyone with limited movement – for instance, a person with sticks or crutches, a mother with young children, someone with a supermarket load of shopping, the elderly. There is minimal luggage space for travellers, and quite a lot of other people can't begin to get on their local bus because the step is too high or there is no provision for wheelchairs. As for getting any help, most buses outside Central London are driver-only operated and he has little time to do more than drive the vehicle and collect the fares.

There are some exceptions. If you live in an area where low entry steps or lifts for wheelchairs have been fitted on some buses, your chances are improved; by national standards you are also pretty lucky, but we must hope that these improvements eventually spread throughout all the bus companies and all the buses.

There are, of course, personal transport schemes for those who cannot use ordinary bus or train services. These include Dial-a-Ride and the many local networks of volunteer drivers who provide transport in their own cars.

In London there has been an encouraging development. London Regional Transport are fitting wheelchair lifts, which can be folded to form a normal step, to all twenty-four of their double-decker Airbus vehicles linking Heathrow Airport and Victoria or Euston. Other main-line railway termini are also being linked to the service by wheelchair-accessible vehicles. This should give people with severe disabilities access to a high-frequency bus service which will make travel less difficult.

All services that help are welcomed, but in the longer term, the aim must be to devise a bus network in which everyone can travel together.

## Trains

Trains are in theory more accessible to all, but your journey may be arduous. British Rail struggle with an inadequate grant to provide services that will make life easier for the disabled. In doing so, however, they are seriously hampered by their many old stations where facilities for the disabled are limited.

The best general advice is to plan your rail journey in advance. Given twenty-four hours' notice, station staff will make what arrangements they can to transfer passengers from the station entrance to the platform.

The trains, too, vary a great deal in accessibility and comfort. Modern suburban and stopping trains are fitted with wide sliding doors and are accessible to wheelchair users – provided they can deal with the external and internal buttons which are sometimes used to operate the doors. Older trains have narrow doorways and wheelchair users have to travel in the guard's van.

Several of our contributors mentioned the difficulty they have had in getting on board trains. The step was not only too high but also too narrow, which meant they had to turn their leading foot at an awkward angle of about ninety degrees before putting their weight on it and hauling themselves up into the train.

# Drive It Yourself

Given that public transport cannot provide for all, it is comforting to be able to report that the possibilities for disabled drivers are now greater than ever before.

You may never have driven a car before, or you may be a disabled driver in need of further help, or a disabled passenger unable to use a conventional vehicle. All kinds of specialist aids and conversions now exist to help give you that essential freedom to travel which can renew people's lives.

Not all conversions are expensive, although some are. It depends on the needs of the individual. Some cars require an almost total refit, and most such one-off conversions are costly, especially where remote-control steering is involved. However, although no two disabilities are quite the same, there are many common solutions which are acceptable to a large number of people – a swivelling car seat, for instance, or a wheelchair hoist and stowage system. In such cases the cost may be relatively small – even though the conversion makes a world of difference.

In the 'Help' section at the end of this book are details of where to go for advice on assessment, finance, rights, benefits and services.

In the five chapters that follow, contributors discuss travelling by train; being pushed in a wheelchair; commuting by car; and car conversions.

# MAINLY ON TRAINS

## Tony Van den Bergh

Tony Van den Bergh, journalist and broadcaster, has had four
hip operations. In 1986 his most recent hip operation was
filmed for television with Tony providing his own live
commentary. Here he talks about his everyday travel
problems, both while working and on holiday; with some
reluctance he observes that he feels safer on the French side
of the Channel.

I put my arthritis down to playing silly sports. After an operation
on an injured knee which I got playing rugby, I started to limp
and walk crookedly. That was the beginning. Over the years the
arthritis has spread, concentrating in my hips, neck, spine and
fingers.

In my work as a journalist I need to travel a lot, and this can
be troublesome. Getting onto buses and trains – anything where
there is a big step up – is difficult and I have to use my arms to
compensate. This has mental repercussions because if I am in
pain I will maybe think, 'This is going to hurt. I shouldn't do it.'
But if I gave in and didn't fight those instincts, I am sure I would
find myself becoming more and more static. Not travelling
would mean not working, and then everything would get steadily
worse.

This is one of the biggest dangers of arthritis. It tends to make
people lazy and they start relying on other people rather than
forcing themselves to act. The older you get, the greater the
danger of this happening.

At the same time, it is a good idea to remain as aware as you
can of your physical limitations. My arthritis was once the cause
of a notable incident on board the Moscow Express. I was
travelling to the USSR as a guest of the trades unions. It was all
very exciting and I had forgotten my pain. Then, halfway to
Moscow, I forgot my age as well. I stood up to put a case on the

rack, my knee caved in under me, and as I fell I grabbed the first handle I could see. Unfortunately it was the Russian version of the emergency cord. I survived only by laying heavy blame on my arthritis!

People say one should take exercise as a way of remaining flexible, but exercise would not agree with me at all. One of my legs is currently 2½ in (6.5 cm) shorter than the other and I wear a built-up shoe. Walking is an effort, especially downhill, however fine the day or however well I am feeling, so once I've dragged myself from one place to the next I feel I have had my exercise and don't need any extra.

As I have got older I have learned to set my natural vanity aside and admit, 'No, I don't think I can do that' when asked if I can perform some physical feat, instead of, as previously, saying yes and suffering afterwards.

My holidays in France often take me to a place where there is a lovely little beach that few people go to. There is no path down to it; you have to scramble down the rock. For years I said, 'Of course I can do it,' when in reality I was terrified the whole way down, especially the last bit where I had to slide on my bottom and hope for a safe landing. I would then spend the last half hour on the beach thinking, 'Oh, God, will I be able to get back up again?'

Luckily, the people I am with now say, 'Don't be silly, you can't do it,' and we don't go there. All the same, it was a blow to my manly pride. Outwardly I may have white hair and hobble about on a stick, but inwardly I am still leading England onto the field at Twickenham.

I cope with travel by planning journeys in advance. On a train I must have a seat, preferably one on the aisle where I can stretch out my leg. If I have to bend it, I soon feel the nerves jerking and it gets very uncomfortable.

Good – by which I mean considerate – design can make an enormous difference to one's comfort while travelling. With trains it starts at the door, as you try to get in.

You know how Olympic weightlifters pause before they make their big effort? They stop, grit their teeth and *will* themselves to succeed, in their case by pulling an enormous barbell upwards above their head. I have to go through a similar self-willing process every time I want to climb on board a train.

I look at that step, so high above the platform, and I *know* my foot will not go up to it. I can't lift it high enough; and yet I have got to. So I concentrate and concentrate, like the weightlifter, then take a deep breath, and with a sudden jerk I lift and push like mad ... and get my foot on the step. Then I rely on the strength of my arms to pull me aboard.

This makes train journeys in Britain never pleasant; it is all such drudgery. In France, by contrast, this problem has been thought about and resolved in a much better way. The steps go up a lot higher, but they start at a reachable level so there is no need to feel discouraged before you begin.

If I want a cup of coffee on a British train, and that rare thing called trolley service is not operating, I feel more than relieved if the person I am with offers to go and get it. For anyone with limited movement, who is perhaps walking with a stick, going through the shaking train is quite a risk. You can very easily be thrown off balance, and just the prospect of that is sometimes terrifying enough. If you have one hand on a stick, the other hand will be fully employed gripping the knobs on top of the seats as you go along. You reach the buffet and buy a finger-scalding container of coffee; then you find you have to drink it on the spot, while swaying this way and that, because it is impossible to carry it back to your seat and drink it there.

In France, again, the carriages are much smoother and better sprung, and you can walk down the train feeling quite safe. That, at least, has been my experience, and it has changed my attitude towards travelling. Now I go abroad with the feeling that the moment I have got across the Channel, I needn't worry any more.

They cater much better in France for the disabled traveller. They have lifts on mainline stations to raise a wheelchair up to the level of the train door; and on the trains there are special carriages for people in wheelchairs and those who accompany them.

Fifteen years ago I wrote a programme on this subject. We went to talk to British Rail and they described some very exciting future plans. Recently they put out a pamphlet which contains almost identical proposals. It is difficult to feel a sense of progress.

# DOOR TO DOOR

If we were allowed just one sourcebook for information about travel for disabled people, we would recommend *Door to Door*. This is a free guide issued by the Department of Transport. It has chapters on:

- Aids and benefits
- Walking and wheelchairs
- Cars
- Taxis
- Individual personal transport schemes
- Buses
- Local trains
- Underground or Metro
- InterCity trains
- Changing stations
- Air travel
- Sea travel
- Coaches
- Community buses and social car schemes
- Local and health authority transport
- Holidays

To obtain a copy, write to Department of Transport and Environment, *Door to Door* Guide, FREEPOST, Victoria Road, South Ruislip, Middlesex HA4 0NZ.

For further information on transport aids, see the 'Help' section at the end of this book.

# WHEELCHAIR FOLLIES

## Laura Mitchell

In her earlier piece, 'Keep Moving', Laura Mitchell talked about helpers in the home and their occasional shortcomings. Here she speaks up for the wheelchair traveller who, perhaps far from home, has to rely on unknown helpers.

Many helpers are good-hearted and will listen to your instructions about how you want to be pushed. Others are less amenable to reason and you wonder why they volunteered at all, unless it was strictly 'for a laugh'. For instance, there is a type of casual helper who thinks it is terribly funny to jiggle you about in your wheelchair. They whirl you round in circles and think they are being entertaining. You, of course, are terrified of being tipped out and find the whole thing exhausting.

By 'casual helper' I mean someone I may ask to help me at a railway station or a conference centre, for example, the kind of place where buildings and departments are spread out a lot and I could not cope on foot. There are no trained people available, so I ask someone who happens to be nearby.

For a start, they don't know how to go up and down pavements. Whenever you make this manoeuvre, you want to be pushed back *into* your chair, not tipped forward out of it. You can cling on, but it is bad for the nerves.

The trouble is, as soon as you get into a wheelchair you become a non-person, subject to all sorts of patronizing 'Does he take sugar?' attitudes and remarks.

In railway stations I dread some of the long slopes leading to and from the platforms. A lot of the porters are very kind, but they are deaf to my fears. I tell them I hate going down ramps.

'Oh, you'll be all right, luv. Don't worry,' they say.

Of course I am not all right. I am hanging on for my life. They don't know what they are talking about.

One simple improvement in this situation would be to fit a seat restraint in every wheelchair. I don't know why it has not been done already. A simple piece of webbing, securely anchored on one side, could be pulled across the body to click or clip into position on the other side. It would make all the difference in the world to people's fears for their safety, especially with respect to being tipped forward and out.*

When I lectured at the London School of Occupational Therapy, they had a system whereby every student spent a whole day pushing a wheelchair with another student in it. Then the first student spent a whole day in the wheelchair. It was a wonderful training. To go out and about, doing the shopping, doing everything from a wheelchair really opened their eyes. Afterwards they would say, 'I never *knew* it was like that.'

Well, it is, and we who do know what it is like must never be afraid to speak up for ourselves. Always try to make others understand.

---

* *Editor's Note:* Restraints are available on quite a few electric wheelchairs, or can be bought separately.

# COMMUTING
# BY CAR

## Peter Nightingale

Peter Nightingale, who drives into London every day to work
(see the chapter 'The Local Government Officer' on page 109),
here discusses his car, a Ford Sierra.

It's an automatic. When I started to drive I could not move my
left leg properly. It was in a funny, bent position and I could not
bend it further or straighten it, so I wasn't able to work the third
pedal on a car. I had to have one I could drive with the right foot
only.

I have had a knee operation since then, but I have always
driven automatics. Because I can't turn my head to look behind
me, I use the wing mirrors a lot and have a wide-angled inside
mirror which I move about to widen my field of vision – for
example, when coming out of a side turning.

I have managed to survive without power steering. I once had
an 1800 which was quite heavy to steer and sometimes, when I
was parked in a tight space, I had to get people to stand outside
the window and pull the wheel round for me.

Generally I find that cars are getting better and better. I
especially like my present car because it is spacious and
comfortable. I have had smaller cars, but if there is less room I
find my shoulders stiffen up.

I can manage public transport – in my case the underground
– for a day or two, but then my hips get too sore. Buses are out for
me. Last year I didn't have the car for a week while it was being
repaired, and I had to use the underground. By the end of the
week I was quite bad – on walking sticks, which is unusual for
me, and feeling so tired and sore that I couldn't do anything in
the evenings except sit down and recover from the journey.

# IN PLACE OF A
# STEERING WHEEL

## Carole Forster

Carole Forster lives in Hampshire. She has had rheumatoid
arthritis/scleroderma for ten years. Within the last year she
has had to give up driving because her arthritis made her
upper arms too weak to steer properly. She consulted Steering
Developments Ltd (see page 155) to see what they suggested.

My arthritis does not fit into any of the more usual categories. It
affects the muscles as well as the joints and some internal
organs such as the throat and lungs. I have joint deformity in my
hands, poor mobility, shoulder pain, and I used to wear a neck
collar when I was driving. I cannot lift things, and my main
problem with driving was to find some form of remote steering
that would relieve me of having to turn a conventional wheel.

I went to be assessed and as a result of that three main
adaptations were proposed: steering would be by means of a
joystick mounted on the driver's door; the handbrake would be
worked electrically by a push-button control; and there would
be a nine-way infra-red switch system to operate controls such
as indicators, horn, wipers, lights, etc. Using the joystick meant
that a lot of the power could be supplied by the wrist rather than
the upper arm, although I still needed to exert some power
through the shoulder.

I had all these adaptations demonstrated to me (partly on the
M1!) and was more than impressed. In fact, I found it quite
inspiring, and for about a month afterwards I was on a high.
Here was a real solution to my problems. I no longer needed to
get depressed thinking I would never be able to drive again. Now
I knew that there was a way.

Unfortunately, practical matters then intervened, i.e., the
cost. Without going into great detail, the cost of converting a new

or fairly young car for me would probably be more than the cost of the basic car. The main reason for the high cost is that I wanted remote-control steering and this costs much more than power steering.* In my case, I needed an estate car with space to take my electric wheelchair and two golden retrievers. After considering various makes and models, I had decided that a Vauxhall Astra Estate would probably suit me best, particularly because of its low loading height.

The total cost, in the region of £15,000, was beyond what I and my husband could manage. That is not to say we won't ever do it, but for the time being a car for me cannot be placed at the top of our financial priorities – unless, that is, we are able to find a further source of help. Meanwhile, I am saving my Mobility Allowance and living in hope.

* *Editor's Note:* Steering Developments Ltd confirm that, at current prices, the cost of remote-control steering starts at £3,750, whereas the cost of power steering starts at £1,000. The former is much more complex, and requires extra back-up and safety features.

# EVERYTHING BAR
# THE WIPERS

## Tanya Raabe

Tanya Raabe is twenty-one and lives near Scarborough in North Yorkshire. She was born with arthrogryphosis multiplex congenita. 'There aren't many of us about,' she says. In terms of mobility, it means her legs and arms do not bend, she cannot bend much from the middle, and her hands are twisted round. How, then, would she achieve her great ambition to drive a car?

I always wanted to drive and when I was seventeen I became even more determined. I don't get pain from the arthritis but my bones are rigid and my muscles have not developed, so I had no chance of driving a conventional car.

I got myself assessed by a local firm and they came up with a solution that involved power steering and some further adaptations. I tried it, but it was not enough. I needed something a lot more radical.

One day I was listening to *Does He Take Sugar?* on the radio. They were talking about cars and driving and said that a mobile unit from Banstead Place Mobility Centre was coming to York. I wrote in and arranged to get myself assessed. When the day came they sat me in a machine to test how strong I was and whether my reflexes were good. A physiotherapist was there to check what movements I was able to perform. I went home and a written assessment soon followed. This satisfied me that I would be able to succeed if I went ahead.

I bought a Ford Escort hatchback from a local dealer. This, by the way, was a special model for the disabled, with extra-long runners for the seat and doors which opened wider. The people at Banstead Place had referred me to Steering Developments Ltd so the dealer drove me down in my car to their factory in

Hemel Hempstead, Hertfordshire. We left the car there for three months while they adapted just about everything bar the wipers to suit me. When I went back, these were the changes they had made:

- It had power-assisted steering and power-assisted brakes.
- The accelerator and the brake were on one lever attached to the left-hand side of the steering wheel. You pull to accelerate and push to brake.
- Also on the same lever was a relay switch to the indicators.
- A steering ball was mounted on the right of the wheel.
- The handbrake was relayed to the right of the driver's seat, and modified to a pull-up/push-down action, mounted at right angles to the floor.
- The automatic gears had the notches taken out of them so I could work the shift. In place of the usual lever I had a long handle.
- The horn was relayed to a pedal on the floor.
- There was a fixed block on which I could rest my left foot, which gave me a more comfortable sitting position.
- The seat was raised 3 in (7.5 cm) at the back and fitted with racing driver seat belts, which are more secure and easier to operate with a magnetic fastening.
- It had an electric window on the driver's side.
- To pull the driver's door shut there was a belt attached to the door from under the steering column.
- There was a wide-angled mirror to give me a better view and save me from turning my head.
- A lever for the dip lights was relayed over the steering column from the left side to the right.

That was it! Apart from the wipers and the switch for the lights, everything had been modified.

I got in the car and took to it straight away. That was in August. In September I began having driving lessons in Scarborough with an ordinary instructor. I took the test in January and passed first time.

# CHOOSING A CAR

The Department of Transport has a useful guide for disabled and elderly people seeking the most convenient car to suit their handicap. Called *Ins and Outs of Car Choice*, it deals with problems of getting in and out of cars with or without a wheelchair or walking aid.

This 42-page guide is available from the Department of Transport and Environment, Publications Sales Unit, Building 1, Victoria Road, South Ruislip, Middlesex HA4 0NZ.

The Department of Transport's Disability Unit runs a free information service on all aspects of transport (public and private) and outdoor mobility for people with disabilities. They welcome inquiries by letter or by telephone. They also conduct full driving assessment tests. You can obtain details from MAVIS, Transport and Road Research Laboratory, Crowthorne, Berkshire RG11 6AU; tel. 0344 779014.

# FAMILY LIFE

## INTRODUCTION

Family life is a complicated structure. It can have about as many strands to it as a cat's cradle, all going this way and that, joining the various members to each other.

The arrival of arthritis in a family can put unexpected strain on this web of relationships. In severe cases everyone, not just the sufferer, must adapt their lives in various ways to accommodate the changes ordered by the disease. It may take time, stretch nerves, and give an enlarged meaning to such virtues as patience, tolerance and generosity.

In this section of the book our contributors look at how arthritis has affected their home life – from the separate points of view of mother, husband and daughter – and describe how they have come to terms with it.

# A MUM WITH
# ARTHRITIS

## Phil Smith

Phil Smith was diagnosed as having rheumatoid arthritis shortly after giving birth to her first child. She thus found herself having to cope with a very painful disease at a time when most mothers need all their strength to cope with their baby and with being a mother. Here she explains what it was like, and how she and her husband Richard have managed since; they now have two children: Christopher, 13, and Lucy, 9. Phil Smith is Chairman of Arthritis Care's 35 Group.

My arthritis is much better than it was. Mainly this is because I now have much better medication and management of the disease, whereas for the first six years it was very active and the medication I was being prescribed by my doctor was not doing the job that it should have been doing.

Once I had got to see a consultant rheumatologist – which took six years because there wasn't one in our area – things became very much better. When Christopher was a baby I used to have five or six bad days a week. Now, on the whole, although I have bad patches, most of the time I have many more good days than bad ones.

The arthritis affects me mainly in my neck, jaw, hands, feet and ankles; from time to time it also affects my knees, hips and elbows. As a child I had all sorts of aches and pains, a stiff neck in particular, and had to miss games for one reason or another. I was continually being taken to the doctor, who said they were growing pains. Fortunately I was able to live a normal life as a teenager – going dancing, staying out late and being told off by my mum, all those things!

I had some more aches and pains later, but it was not until I was expecting Christopher that I began to get a lot of pain in one arm and then couldn't use it at all. I hadn't been pregnant before, so I didn't know what to expect.

The birth was perfectly normal: everything was fine. I came home after ten days feeling OK. Christopher was three weeks old when suddenly it happened. It was like getting a very bad dose of flu. I went to bed at eight o'clock one evening; at ten o'clock I couldn't move. My husband had to take me to the toilet, feed me, give me a drink. He called the doctor, who thought it was overtiredness. After some further examinations, which got nowhere, I mentioned that my mother had arthritis and could there be any connection? I was sent for a blood test and x-rays, and then it was diagnosed: rheumatoid arthritis.

Diagnosis can take much longer so in a way I was lucky. The problem then was to find a way of relieving the pain which would not get in the way of my looking after Christopher. It was a very difficult time.

One of the big changes I had to get used to was how long it took me to do everything. I don't think it can be a truly common feature, but a lot of arthritis sufferers I know are fastidious people. I was the same: everything had to have its place; everything had to be done in the right order. If it was Monday, it was windows; that was me. Now here I was with this new baby I had been desperate to have – and I couldn't even pick him up out of his cot.

Before I could do anything for him I had to hold him to me, haul him out of the cot and then sort of shuffle into my bedroom and drop him on the double bed. My husband took the odd day off from work to help me, but most days I was on my own with Christopher until Rich came home in the evening. Then he would look after us. I also had some very good friends who came in from time to time, but I wanted to be independent no matter how long it took. And it did take hours.

To do the washing, I had a twin-tub machine and a boiler for nappies. Disposable nappies weren't really to the fore in those days, so you bleached nappies and boiled them. At times it was very frustrating. The boiler used to boil over, and then I couldn't get the nappies out of it. We finally saved up enough money to buy an automatic washing machine. Christopher was about eight months old by then, and for us it was a turning point. We should have done it in the beginning but we couldn't afford it.

Having got the automatic washing machine, it was no longer a problem to wash nappies. They went on the boil and that was it. But – I couldn't always peg them out on the line. That meant either having them indoors, dripping on an airer, or keeping up the struggle with clothes pegs until, after an awful lot of effort, I had them over the line and pegged in place.

All the housework was like that. It took ages, and I was tired when I started. Halfway through I'd think, 'Oh, gosh, I wish I hadn't started this.' But you have to do it.

Giving Christopher a bath was very difficult. Either it had to wait until Rich came home at night or I would tackle it myself, with Christopher in a baby bath in the big bath and me sitting on a chair trying to support him. On the days when I couldn't manage that, he had to have a top-to-tail wash.

I did not have enough help. I know a lot of mums in a similar situation to myself who did not and do not get help when they most need it. When Christopher was a few weeks old a health visitor came round: 'Are you all right? Is he all right? Are you coping?' – as they say to every young mum. She knew that I had rheumatoid arthritis but she did not have any idea about what might be available to help me – equipment to raise the cot and the carrycot, for example, or things to help in the bathroom. No suggestions were made whatsoever. If I had known then what I know now, life would have been a lot easier. But I didn't.

Looking back, it is amazing what you can make yourself do. Take dressing, for instance. I had this thing about Christopher wearing socks; my baby had to wear socks. It took me an hour sometimes to put them on. You learn as you go along. As time goes by you accept that you don't have to do this and you don't really need that; yet at the same time there are lots of things that are essential. Babies have to be fed, washed, exercised – and played with.

As soon as Christopher started to crawl, I knew there would be trouble. He was not an easy child anyway, and that stage was a nightmare; we both experienced a great deal of frustration. Getting down on the floor with him was agony for me, so I tried to adapt. I found I was telling him off more than I wanted to, but I had to rely on words to restrain him because I couldn't keep up with him physically. I could not chase after him and retrieve him from the fireplace, or the wires ... or the Christmas tree.

That sort of crisis always happens suddenly, out of nowhere. One moment the Christmas tree was standing there, the next it was starting to topple, and it was going to fall on my son. What should I do? An able-bodied mum might have managed to dash across the room and grab the tree in time. All I could do was stagger towards Christopher and hope I could pull him out of the way. I got to him just before the tree did. He was safe, and that was fine. He was what mattered, not the tree. All the same, if I could have stopped the tree from falling, I would not have had baubles and bits of decoration all over the place which took me hours to clear up. Incidents like that, which most able-bodied people take in their stride, can get you down if you aren't able to deal with them quickly. If you aren't careful, they can make you depressed.

## And What About the Husband?

I was very concerned about my husband, and I think what I felt must be a fear with many women who have arthritis. He has always been very supportive, and I have been very lucky in that respect; but in the early days I remember thinking, 'What am I going to do if he leaves me?' I didn't want him to go – of course I didn't – but if he had decided to leave us, I would have understood.

The husband of someone with arthritis has a lot of pressure on him. He comes in the door after a long day at work and he does not know what he is going to find. It may be all right: she may have felt OK and been able to manage. But supposing she had had a bad day, which had been a real struggle to get through – what then? I can imagine husbands standing outside the door and thinking, 'What's going to face me tonight?'

If it's not been a good day, the husband will have to take over and be Mum for the rest of the evening: clear up the mess, look after the kids, prepare the vegetables, cook the meal, wash up – the lot. At least, that is what Rich did for me – and still does.

## The Children and Me

The decision to have another child was purely selfish on my part. I am an only child and I did not want my son to be one. I had always wanted other children. So when Christopher was one year old we decided to try for another baby in case my arthritis grew worse with time and reached a point where we would not be able to consider having a second child. This plan didn't work out immediately; in fact, Christopher was nearly four when Lucy was born. I later discovered that this could have been caused by the arthritis: arthritic flare-ups tend to suppress your fertility.

The delay was a blessing in disguise, however, because by then Christopher was able to help me in the house. The only thing that put him out at all when he saw his little sister for the first time was – she was not green! He had wanted a green baby.

After Lucy was born I felt fine, or better than usual, anyway. Then, when she was five months old, the arthritis came back with a vengeance and life was a big struggle again. How we all managed to come through I am not quite sure. When I think of all the washing, shopping, cooking, bathing, housework, plus the pain and fatigue which at times seemed endless, I can only think that I managed because of the children. They were my objectives in life, and looking after them is what I set myself to do.

Today our family life is lovely. Both the children are very independent, as they probably need to be. I have felt much better in myself since I began seeing the rheumatologist and getting better medication. Also, the day came when I did not need to look after the children *all* the time. Young children want physical contact with Mum: they want to sit on your lap; they want to be cuddled; they have to be carried up and down stairs when they are tiny. I was quite relieved when we got past those stages and they were able to do things for themselves. Then they began to go to school and that gave me a very welcome rest in the mornings.

Perhaps I let them find their own way sooner than most mothers would choose. I suspect that is typical of a mum with arthritis. I don't ask them to do a lot for me – in fact, I have to nag them rotten sometimes – but if I am feeling bad they will recognize this and rally round. They are very good. When I am back on my feet again, they are just like all kids – pushing their luck as far as they can!

# LOOKING AFTER BECKY

## Shirley Poulton

Becky Poulton is three and has chronic juvenile arthritis. The first signs appeared when she was three months old. Diagnosis took ten months and she then underwent long and intensive treatment, as a result of which she is now making a good recovery. Her mother, Shirley Poulton, recalls here what happened.

Becky is very good at the moment. Her ankles and knees are weak so she can't do any jumping movements, and she wears built-up boots with inserts to give her extra support. She can just about get up the stairs on her bottom, but she can't walk up them. She is awkward with her hands because both her wrist joints are affected.

She looks a lot better than she used to. The medicines that she is on now, and the steroids that she has had in the past, have taken away the inflammation. Unless you look quite closely, you can't see that there is much wrong except that she is very thin.

She is very bright and needs a lot of stimulation. People have said that children with physical handicaps are brighter in other respects, to make up for the things they lose out on. She works her way through games and toys very quickly, and we constantly have to get her new ones. It costs a fortune, but we think it is important to keep her occupied mentally.

When the arthritis began, she had a swollen finger and a swollen toe on her right side. It was ten months before arthritis was diagnosed. At first they suspected meningitis, then gastro-enteritis, and Becky had to have numerous tests in hospital before these could be eliminated. Then we took her to see a consultant rheumatologist who said immediately that it was arthritis. One of the reasons why diagnosis had taken so long was that she did not have the typical Still's rash, as it is called, although it has appeared since.

She has had what they call bone damage, which has made her knees slightly distorted. Her right leg won't go completely straight. She was in plaster and splints for months while they worked to straighten it. Now she is back in splints at night because the knee is getting bad again.

She walks confidently now, but it took us months to get her to take her first steps on her own. She took those on 6 May 1985, at half-past one in the afternoon [*laughter*]: she walked from the television over to the settee. In the last couple of months she has tried crawling on her knees as well as walking. She never crawled as a baby because it was too painful.

She used to scream all the time. We couldn't cuddle her because that squeezed the joints and made it worse, and for months we just didn't know what was going on or what we should do. Her joints were so sore it was agony for her just to have her bottom lifted up so I could put her nappy on. If I touched her ankle she screamed and screamed.

Then she had an intensive hydrotherapy course and it was the best thing that has happened to her. For three months she was in hospital receiving hydrotherapy twice a day, plus normal physiotherapy. We still take her twice a week for hydrotherapy, and we are sure that she would not be walking now if it had not been for this treatment.

At home she had to have physiotherapy three times a day – morning, noon and night. She needed to wear leg splints, which we were always adjusting because they kept slipping down. She had wrist splints, too, and these had to be checked regularly to make sure they didn't make her sweat or rub and make her sore. In addition, she had a brace for her neck because that was also affected. On top of all this we had to get her to take her medication. It was all a lot of hard work, but now we can see how essential it was. If we had sat back and waited for her to 'grow out of it', she would never have made any progress – and in fact would have got worse.

Most of the time it was a matter of trying to keep her happy. She could hardly move by herself – all she could do was shuffle about on her bottom. We used to give her something to help her get to sleep, and once she was asleep she wasn't too bad; but if she woke up she would be terribly stiff. There was a spell when she woke up every night and her neck was so stiff she couldn't move it. The stiffness would last for a couple of hours. She still wakes up stiff, but now it's usually worse if it's after a short sleep, like an afternoon nap.

It took me ages to come to terms with the fact that she had arthritis. My husband managed, but at first I couldn't believe it. I associated arthritis with older people. My grandmother had had it, but that seemed to make it all the more difficult to understand.

Fortunately Becky is much better now. She has the occasional flare-up and has to go into hospital, usually for a week, to have it brought under control. She is getting generally stronger all the time, though, and one of the things we must try to do now is fatten her up. We also have to have her eyes tested regularly, because of the arthritis; she has had conjunctivitis in the past so we do this every three months.

She is down to go to the local nursery school shortly before her fourth birthday. She is brighter than most children of her age and should find school work no problem. On the social side, however, she is very shy and of course she is not able to take part in the rough and tumble of playground life. That is a worry because, as we know from one or two experiences, young children like to rush about; they don't look where they are going, and it is all too easy to knock Becky over. If she has a fall she gets a lot of pain and it takes her a long time to get over it.

Looking ahead, we will also have to be careful about her mixing with other children because of the dangers of infection. Once arthritis was diagnosed, she was not able to have any more of the usual vaccinations, so if the slightest thing is going around, down she goes with a temperature. When this happens, her joints start swelling and her blood pressure goes up – and this involves her heart. She has a slight heart murmur which has to be watched: in the beginning they thought it might be a hole in the heart, but the murmur has steadied down a lot since then, and she has regular check-ups. As a result of all this, though, even a simple cold can cause an awful lot of complications. One of the hazards of going to school is that, in their first year, children are liable to catch anything and everything. We hope and pray that we are able to make Becky strong enough to fight these infections when they crop up.

We have come a long way in three years.

# AIDS FOR CHILDREN

Helpful items on display at the Disabled Living Foundation's Aids Centre in London include the following:

## Mobility
- Standing and walking frames; tricycles
- Pushchairs; electric wheelchairs

## Seating
- Toilet seats with extra support
- Bathing aids
- Children's chairs and tables
- Car seats; head protectors

## Eating and drinking
- Drinking cups and feeding aids

For further information, see the 'Help' section at the end of the book.

# 'THE MAN WHO DOESN'T HAVE ARTHRITIS'

## Alan Rogers

Alan Rogers is a senior BBC executive in charge of the
Magazine branch of Current Affairs Radio. Among the
programmes in his care are *Does He Take Sugar?* and *You
and Yours*. He began showing symptoms of arthritis at the
age of nineteen or so. In his early forties he underwent two hip
replacement operations and he now regards himself as
largely free of the disease. Here he talks about his on/off
experience of arthritis and its effects on his family life.

I can totally forget that I have arthritis for a lot of the time, but
I have to accept that with my tin hips I find it difficult to do
certain things: getting in and out of a car or a boat, for example
– awkward manoeuvres like that where the seat is low. Moving
furniture is also difficult; I can lift things all right, but I have
some arthritis in my hands so I cannot grip very hard.

It has become a standing joke at home. I go around claiming
there is nothing wrong with me, and then my wife Jenny sees me
struggling to move a chair. 'Oh, yes,' she says, 'I can see you
haven't got arthritis.'

It is nevertheless true that I feel very much better and can do
much more than I could when my arthritis was at its peak. That
was before I had my hip operations and when I was walking
about with a built-up shoe and a stick.

I began to have symptoms when I was nineteen or twenty: I
had pain in the hips and found that I was limping. Arthritis was
not diagnosed at that point because the pain went away for some
years and did not return until I was in my early thirties. It was

then diagnosed as ankylosing spondylitis. I subsequently went in for a lot of exercises and physiotherapy, which made it much better.

Curiously enough, the day it was diagnosed I happened to be watching a regional television programme. They were excavating a Saxon burial ground, and the archaeologist picked up a long, bent piece of bone. 'This is some poor Saxon's backbone,' he said. 'All bent, as you can see. He suffered from a thing we call ankylosing spondylitis. He must have died in great pain.'

That's wonderful, I thought. All the encouragement I need! But in actual fact, today's drugs and treatments make everything so much easier for the patient. My condition improved considerably, and it was not until several years later that I began to get a lot of hip pain. In time I had to wear a built-up shoe because one hip had clenched up and made that leg about 1½ in (3.75 cm) shorter than the other one.

For about a year I was fairly severely disabled. Then I went to the Rheumatology Department of Wanstead Hospital, Essex, and they recommended me to have both hips replaced. I was taking a painkiller for much of that time, which provided some relief, but I still felt stiff and weakened by the disease.

## New Hips, New Life

Since the operations, my life has been transformed. I now live a normal, active life. I can play with my kids, go sailing, do all kinds of things that would have been impossible before.

On the debit side, I have a swollen leg and ankle and two swollen knees – a classic consequence of ankylosing spondylitis. I have some stiffness in my hands and neck, which limits arm and head movements to some extent. I will also have to take drugs regularly for the rest of my life. But I regard all these as trivial matters when set beside the quality of life which I am now able to lead.

I should perhaps mention one problem I had over drugs. For some years I had been taking a particular anti-inflammatory drug and it had worked very well for me. Then my wife and I began to consider having children. Originally we had thought we would not have children, but after we had been married for ten years we began to change our minds.

I remembered someone saying that the drug I was taking could infect the male sperm and cause damaged babies. I checked this out with the manufacturers, asking them for any research papers they had. I got a whole load of literature from them addressed to 'Dr Alan Rogers'! I read it and, sure enough, discovered that the drug can infect the sperm. I saw my doctor about it and switched to another drug. Later my wife gave birth to two boys and they are both fine.

If I had stayed on the first drug, the risk would not have been a great one, but it did exist. I certainly believe that people should read or find out as much as possible about the drugs they take.

My boys, Luke and Owen, are now eleven and nine. I can play football and cricket with them, take them sailing, go cycling. I can't run great distances, but I manage to play some badminton – it is one of those games where, if you are devious and tactically minded, you can avoid running about too much.

For their part, the boys look after me. They are perfectly aware that I do not like reaching into awkward corners to pick something up; so they do it for me. My wife, too, has been marvellously tolerant. When I was going through my painful period, before the operations, it was tempting to struggle on at the office through the day, then go home with no energy left and be grumpy for the rest of the evening. That is something one has to watch. I am grateful I have a wife who can put up with me.

# GROWING UP TOGETHER

## Janet Flower

Janet Flower began to suffer from rheumatoid arthritis when she was three. She is now twenty-seven and lives with her parents and two brothers in East London. She works as a secretary-receptionist, drives her own car, and is a regional contact for Arthritis Care's 35 Group. She and her mother discuss here the problems of having arthritis in the family.

**Janet** Arthritis affects all my joints and I have had both hips replaced. Although people like me may end up adapting to their arthritis, I don't think they ever get used to it. I still feel there is a normal person inside me waiting to come out.

When you are diagnosed, the other members of the family have to learn to cope as well. It surprises me that, even today, they do not receive much advice about what to expect. In my case, I still find I get frustrated and annoyed, and I tend to take it out on the people I live with. It can be hard on someone who is trying to help you, perhaps by opening a door, if you turn round and snap at them, 'I can do it!'.

**Mrs Flower** It is difficult for the parent always to know what is best. Probably they don't know what it is like to have arthritis and so they don't know what the child is feeling. I used to be strict with Janet about her exercises. I'd say to her, 'You do those exercises. You've got to.' 'I don't want to,' she'd say. 'You've got to!' I'd tell her.

**Janet** And then we'd be having a battle. Obviously I didn't understand what was going on at the time, but as I grew up I began to see how difficult it was for parents to find the right course to take. They can be wrong if they are over-protective and don't take the children anywhere or let them deal with new and possibly difficult experiences; and they can be wrong if they give them too much independence, so they become hard or bitter about what they see as neglect.

I still don't find it easy to cope with my problems; it depends on whether it's a good day or a bad day, and it changes all the time. So how can I expect my parents to know how I feel?

**Mrs Flower**  You have to try to make them independent. That goes for all your children. I found it very difficult at first to come to terms with my child being disabled, and I worried all the time about looking after her. Now I get worried if she wants to go off somewhere, say to a pop concert. My first reaction is: 'Oh, no! All those stairs, all those people. She only needs to be pushed over . . . .' I get over that, but then I say to her, 'How are you going to get there? You're not driving. Surely you're not going in your car all across London?' 'Yes, I am,' she says.

**Janet**  It's just as well she does worry sometimes, because I don't always think things out for myself. I say 'yes' to an invitation, then need reminding that I don't know how to get there.

Sometimes I can be a bit too independent by going to work when I am having a bad day. I struggle through at the office, but when I get home I've had enough. I'm tired, so I let my hair down, moan, shout at the dog. It's not fair, really, but I suppose everyone's a bit like that.

**Mrs Flower**  The thing is, if you're at home with your family, with the people you know best of all, you *can* let yourself go.

**Janet**  In a way you want people to notice and you want a bit of sympathy; but at the same time you don't want the fuss. With my brothers, Roy and Alan, it's a little bit different. They have been good for me in that with them I learnt to stand up for myself. When I was a child I had to find ways of not having my toys snatched off me by them because I couldn't run after them. As we got older, they became more helpful and now they look after me if I need something.

At the same time they can't be thinking of me all the time, and I shouldn't expect them to. A bone of contention at the moment, for example, is the shower. It's one of those where the spray is fixed to a pole so you can push it up and down to suit yourself. Sometimes they leave it right at the very top, way out of reach for me. If I'm feeling a bit touchy, I'll think, 'Oh, no. How long have I had arthritis? Why don't they know I can't reach that far?' So I shout down the stairs, 'Who's gone and left the shower like that – *again*?' 'Oh, stop moaning,' they say – which is about right sometimes. It has to be give and take on both sides.

# LUPUS IN THE FAMILY

## Cheryl Marcus

Cheryl Marcus was twenty-one when she was diagnosed as
having lupus, or systemic lupus erythematosus (SLE). This is
a systemic disease which can cause arthritis as well as many
other distressing symptoms. Despite suffering many severe
flare-ups, she has managed, with help and support, to raise a
family. Here she talks about her experience of the disease and
its effect on family life, and about her work for the Lupus
Group which she founded and which is now part of Arthritis
Care.

I had been complaining to my doctor for quite a while about
aching joints; I felt tired a lot of the time and had been running
temperatures. He said he thought it was growing pains. I was
engaged to be married, and as the wedding came nearer I was
told that my troubles were wedding nerves. Deep down I thought
it was something else but I didn't know what.

One of the main symptoms of lupus is a rash caused by
sunbathing. We went to Portugal for our honeymoon. It was the
first time I had been exposed to strong sunlight. I went out to
sunbathe, came out in a terrible rash, my joints began to ache,
and we had to come home as quickly as we could.

I was luckier than most in that my father was a doctor and he
was able to refer me to the correct person straight away, so I had
a fairly prompt diagnosis. A lot of sufferers get really ill before
they are diagnosed. They go through the trauma of not knowing
what's wrong and beginning to think they are psychologically
unbalanced or abnormal in some awful way. Lupus *is* such a
strange disease, and may appear in any organ of the body, so
there is no obvious pattern for an ordinary person to go by.

Even today I meet people who have been on the verge of
having a kidney transplant without knowing they had lupus.
They had been labelled 'kidney patient' without anyone realiz-

ing that something else was causing the problem. When I was diagnosed there were doctors walking around at the end of my bed consulting a book to find out what lupus was; they didn't know. Not that the books of that time were very reliable: anyone looking up lupus would be informed it was a fatal disease. It *can* be, but this is very rare and should not happen if proper treatment is given.

In my case, my joints seized up so badly that I was in a wheelchair. I had severe circulatory problems, which seriously affected my fingers and toes. I suffered convulsions, and it was not clear whether they were caused by the lupus or by the steroid drugs I had been taking. I was transferred between a neurology ward (for my head), a rheumatology ward (for my joints) and a haematology ward (for my circulation). At first they didn't really know what to do with me.

Today the process of diagnosis is much quicker and surer, and the treatment is better. Doctors are, or should be, better informed. Nowadays a patient with symptoms of lupus should be referred to hospital for a DNA blood test, which is a straightforward way of diagnosing the disease. However, I still receive reports about doctors not being sufficiently aware of this test, which means that some patients are still not diagnosed as early as they should be. Now that we have the Lupus Group, we attack doctors regularly with mailing shots to help increase their awareness.

Not every lupus sufferer has convulsions – in fact, it is not all that common – but it is worth mentioning that they are distressing for those who see them. I didn't know anything about mine until I woke up in hospital, but my husband thought I was dead. I collapsed suddenly, went very rigid, my eyes rolled back and blood came out of my mouth. This was because I had bitten my tongue, so now they know that one of the first things to do is to pull the tongue forwards. My elder son has also seen it happen, and I know he found it frightening.

The circulatory problem meant that if I cut my finger it went very messy. This was because in lupus the body's immune system is upset and antibodies in the blood turn against your own tissues.

To look at I was quite a sight. I was covered in a rash, I lost my hair completely, and my weight went up to 13 st (82.5 kg) because of the amount of steroids I was being given. A lot of people were scared to come near me, and my son was not allowed to visit me because we were worried about the effect it might have on him. It was a tough time, and I am not sure that I could have done much to reassure him.

One of the problems of lupus is that you can become very isolated. It is difficult to explain to your friends what you've got, because it has a strange name and a strange nature and they probably haven't heard of it before. You look terrible, so you'd rather they didn't see you anyway, and the word goes around that you are in hospital with this 'thing' but that it's best not to visit just now because you are a frightening sight.

This at least is something we can help with in our Group. We understand this loneliness and can tell people that it doesn't have to go on for ever. And we can put them in touch with consultants who can really help them.

My various conditions followed one another over a period of time. There had also been the problem of pregnancy. As soon as I was diagnosed we were told that the outlook for a successful pregnancy was not good. We decided to take a chance and not wait, in case I got worse. I became pregnant immediately and had my first child within a year of getting married.

## Parents to the Rescue

During the pregnancy I was fine, but in the delivery stage and after my son was born the lupus came back with a vengeance. It soon became clear that I would not be able to bring him up myself. I would have to spend a lot of time in hospital, and when I was at home I would not be able to cope.

Martin, my husband, and my parents got together. He sold our house, my parents sold their flat, and together they bought one big house and converted it into two flats. My parents lived upstairs, and my husband and the baby were downstairs. This gave Martin a degree of independence, and at the same time he didn't have to worry about getting someone in to care for the baby: my parents did all that, as well as the cooking and cleaning.

I have been exceptionally lucky to have such an understanding husband, and parents who were prepared to change their way of life to help us. I remember feeling very guilty as I lay in bed in hospital and the months went by. I suppose that was natural.

I suffered badly from the disease for five or six years. In America they were doing much more research into lupus than they were in Britain. My father wrote to an American hospital and they said they would like to see me if I went over there. Then it was decided that I was too ill to travel. We seemed to be getting nowhere when a letter arrived to tell us that a doctor who had studied lupus in America was coming to England to work at Hammersmith Hospital in London.

This was fantastic news. Even so, when I went to Hammersmith Hospital I did not really feel there was much that the specialist could do for me. I was in a wheelchair; I couldn't walk; I was obese; I was bald; I was in continual severe pain. But he had other ideas. He said, 'You're not going to leave this hospital until you are out of that wheelchair.'

From that day my life changed. I was in hospital for a long time but at last I began to make progress. My drugs were altered so I took less steroids; a lot of the treatment was experimental, but the specialist was determined that things would work out in the end. Slowly my weight began to reduce, my hair started to grow again, and I moved onto a walking frame and then to crutches. I underwent many operations during this time, but eventually I was able to go home. I still needed nursing and had to do a lot of physiotherapy, but after two or three years I was leading a comparatively normal life – at home.

When I reached that stage, we decided in the family that Martin and I could now set up our own home and my parents could do the same and enjoy an independent life. This is what we did; my parents moved to a place not far away, so they could help if needed, and Martin and I began to live as we do today. I have daily help with the housework, and recently I have been driving a car.

Four years ago I desperately wanted to have another child. I was warned that things could go wrong, but I felt it was better to try and fail rather than not make an attempt. I saw a gynaecologist at Hammersmith Hospital who said that if we were prepared to take the gamble, he would see us through it. When I became pregnant I went into hospital and stayed there. At seven months, because the baby had stopped growing and the lupus was beginning to show signs of returning, they did a Caesarian. Jonathan was born, weighing 2½ lb (1 kg). He had to fight to live; he was in intensive care for a long time, but he survived. When I got him home he was three months old.

So, I have two sons, aged thirteen and four. There's a big gap between them but I wouldn't have it any other way. In that time medical opinion has changed, and in general it is now not thought so risky for a woman with lupus to have a baby. However, after Jonathan they did say to me, 'Don't do it again.'

Today my health, like so many people with lupus, is unpredictable. I need to have replacement joints in my shoulders but these are not in a good enough state to receive them. In the meantime I am having operations to build up the bone and make it possible for me to have replacements. I suffer from migraines, which I assume are connected with the earlier convulsions; these are very severe and I have to go to bed for forty-eight hours. They are antisocial as well as painful, and make me wary of arranging outings or meetings too far ahead. I get very tired, and sleep for two hours every afternoon. I also have other problems because of my poor circulation.

Luckily, I have some good friends who take it in turns to pick up Jonathan from school. My elder son, Daniel, is old enough to know what is going on, and by and large we have adapted very well as a family to my condition. Thank goodness my husband has been able to adapt as well. Sport is probably what has kept him going. By playing a lot of golf, tennis and table tennis he has been able to give himself an independent life outside the family instead of being tied all the time to a sick wife.

## Nice Round Faces

I now look extremely healthy. A lot of lupus people do. We have nice round faces, some rounder than others – an effect of the steroids we take.

I have pink rosy cheeks. This is because I have a rash, which I cover up with powder.

I look suntanned. This is because I take an anti-malarial drug which tends to make the skin look yellow.

Looks are truly deceptive. I know a lot of lupus people get very frustrated when people tell them how plump and well they look, when all the time they know it is because they are on extra steroids and in fact are feeling grotty.

# The Lupus Group

I started the Lupus Group, and we now have 2,500 members and are growing fast. We have eighteen regional groups in Britain and we are linking up with the Lupus Foundation in the United States, and through them with national groups in other countries.

Our Group began when I was in a London hospital (not the Hammersmith) and feeling very ill and alone. I thought, 'There must be just *one* other person out there who has lupus.' I couldn't write my own letters, so I got a friend to write to Radio London saying that her friend had this strange disease called lupus, and if anyone else had it, could they write to her at the hospital. Next thing, Radio London came round to the hospital and let me broadcast my own message.

I had a reply from a girl who lived in Hertfordshire. She was able to come and see me in hospital, and it helped me such a lot to meet her and be able to talk about it. Then my message was broadcast on the regional network and the numbers began to creep up: ten, twenty, and after a year or so I had gathered about fifty people.

When I was at home again, the numbers grew to such an extent that it became too much for me to cope with. I approached Arthritis Care, because we had the rheumatic factor in common, and they agreed to take us on under their umbrella. Since then we have formed another body, which works in parallel with our caring and welfare group. This is called the British SLE Aid Group, which raises funds for research at the hospitals which have lupus patients.

A lot more research needs to be done – but now at least we feel that we are getting somewhere.

# SOCIAL LIFE

## INTRODUCTION

Social life can mean anything from finding a partner to going out in the evening. Many people with arthritis have to face extra difficulties because the generally able-bodied world they live in is not always geared to their needs. Opportunities for meeting people may arise less frequently than they wish, and problems of transport and facilities can pose discouraging barriers.

However, the four contributors to this section of the book are united in their determination to keep on trying. For them the effort is always worthwhile; the idea of not going anywhere is something they firmly reject.

# A SHORTAGE OF MEN

## Rosemary Sutcliff

Novelist Rosemary Sutcliff likes the company of men, but finds them much harder to meet than women.

It is beginning to be accepted that the disabled have emotions. Today it is not all that unusual to find a disabled couple, or one disabled person and one able-bodied person, in love with each other. When I was young it was unheard of.

It must still be difficult for two such people to manage – and difficult for them to meet each other in the first place. This lack of opportunity applies to plenty of people other than the disabled. Any woman on her own has very few opportunities for meeting men, whether they are attached or unattached.

Your women friends ask you in for coffee when their husbands are out. If they are having a dinner party they don't ask you at all, because that would mean finding an unattached male. I share this problem with several women friends who are either unmarried or divorced – we just do *not* meet men. Being disabled simply makes it even harder.

If, like me, you enjoy the company of men, this is a great disappointment. Being with women all the time can give you a blinkered, feminine-only viewpoint. I do meet a certain number of men with whom I talk shop. They are writers, or people in publishing, or librarians or visiting professors. I enjoy these conversations very much, but they are not as interesting as talking to someone from another walk of life who happens to be a man.

I have another problem: I am not a herd animal, and I don't like occasions such as drinks parties. If you are in a wheelchair, people either talk above your head or bend down and put their face next to yours, which is quite off-putting.

We 'singles' in the wheelchairs have a lot to hope for. We have reached a stage where our existence has become respectable, but our presence still seems rather inconvenient.

# A LONG TIME
# SINGLE

## Peter Nightingale

Peter Nightingale puts in a lot of spare-time work for Arthritis Care's 35 Group. He knows it is not easy for young people with arthritis to form independent relationships.

Everything takes longer if you have arthritis, which is why at the age of thirty-two I am still living at home with my mum and dad.

This is not unusual among the people with arthritis that I know, but it is unusual among the population as a whole. For many it goes back to when they were about fourteen to sixteen. Other kids were going out in the evenings and meeting new people, but they weren't. I never used to mix with anyone after school. I went to a single-sex school, I was picked up in the afternoon and taken home, and that was it. My friends were getting on with their social growing-up bit, but I missed out on that.

Later, a lot of young people want to leave home and share a flat with their mates. For someone who is going to need help, it is that much harder to make the jump. You don't want to impose on others, so then you start to think it would be safer to stay at home. If you need a high bed, for instance, you might worry whether you'd be able to get one in a furnished flat. It's probably not a major difficulty, in fact, but at the time you may think it is, and this may make you decide to stay at home.

The result is that you need more time to grow up and mature. I am engaged now, and my fiancée, who also has arthritis, is twenty-seven and also still lives at home. A lot of the people I know who have arthritis are young women in their late twenties and early thirties who live at home. Rheumatoid arthritis affects more women than men – about three to one.

We are hoping to get married in 1987, by which time I will have saved enough to put down a deposit on a house. I expect it will be difficult for us at first, but it has worked out well so far.

When you are on your own you have to be resilient. It's easy to persuade yourself into thinking that no-one will ever be attracted to you, and to let yourself be too self-conscious. Even now, I ought to wear splints on my hands every day, but I don't, especially if I am going out. I don't want people looking at me. Probably they aren't looking at me, but I may think they are. It's something you have to be careful about.

# GIRLS ON TOP

## Kay James and Kata Kolbert

Someone said of them: 'They've got an awful lot of nerve, those two. They are punk rockers. They wear splints on their legs and fishnet stockings, and they go around in wheelchairs. Nutters really. I wish them the best of luck.'

Kay James and Kata Kolbert are in their twenties. Both contracted rheumatoid arthritis in childhood. They met in hospital and found they had so many interests in common that they decided they must leave home and find a flat together. It was a long struggle even to get that far, but they made it. Now they have other ambitions.

**Kata**  We are in wheelchairs, but it's no big deal that we can't walk. You get used to it. Before I moved in here I could walk about a bit, around the flat, and stand up to cook, but now I have to stay in my wheelchair. This has happened before; it fluctuates. For me to try to walk now would give me excruciating agony. I can cope in the wheelchair, so it's not all that important.

**Kay**  Earlier in the year I had to go into hospital for three weeks. The doctor thought it was because of having moved into this flat. It was the first time I had lived away from home and he said I'd overdone it, so I went in for a rest. I was completely worn out. Hopefully it won't happen again. I think it was like a warning, so now I take it a bit easier if I'm feeling tired.

**Kata**  Getting into this flat was the biggest hassle we have ever had in our lives. We met in hospital and immediately became friends. We were interested in things, like writing and music, which other people thought were weird, but that didn't put us off. When we went home it was difficult to meet because I lived in Slough with my parents and Kay lived around here [in Leytonstone, East London]. We had horrendous telephone bills. Sometimes we went and stayed with each other, but that was quite intermittent.

After about two years of that we realized that all the things we wanted to do required independence. That meant being together, preferably in London, because whenever we went out to a club or a concert from Slough we had to get minicabs there and back and it was costing a fortune. Even if I came to stay with Kay and her parents I still had to pay the fares. We decided, if we were ever going to do anything, from social life to more serious ambitions, we needed to be together.

We started with a list of about a hundred addresses from housing associations. We slowly ploughed through them and got our names put on lists, most of which would have meant waiting ten years or so – either that or we didn't qualify. There was one women's association that had housing, but you had to be over twenty-five, and they were worried, because some parts of the house were shared, about the noise we'd make. Others said we weren't important because we weren't a couple getting married. Also, I wasn't a London resident. We couldn't get any priority.

Then someone told us to try the Greater London Council. We wrote to Ken Livingstone and he suggested we should apply for council housing, putting us in touch with the relevant people. This was a big breakthrough because we had assumed we didn't stand a chance with the local authorities: after all, we were still living at home with our parents and they weren't actually throwing us out.

It was still a struggle because I had to be transferred from one authority, Chiltern Council, to another, Waltham Forest. That took ages because they wouldn't believe that I really wanted to do it. I had to go to meet committees to try to convince them.

Six months later, however, I got the transfer, and then we were told we would be considered as joint tenants for whatever place came up. Fortunately the next stage was quicker, and after about three months we were offered this flat. We took it straightaway, but then they spent another eighteen months messing about with the conversion work.

**Kay** They had to knock down walls to make the bathroom bigger, redo the kitchen, and make the doors wider for our wheelchairs. Even so, weeks went by when nothing happened. We later found out, after we moved in, that our file had been lost for six months.

They had the floorboards up three times. The first time was because they hadn't checked properly and there was a stream underneath the building, which flooded. Then, when they'd skipped over something else, they had to have the boards up again. They also had to send all the kitchen units back because the first lot delivered were standard size, instead of special ones at wheelchair height.

**Kata**   All this time we were waiting to move in. Whenever we asked what was happening, we met this blank wall. I was in trouble with my family as well, because they were moving to Devon but had to wait for me to move in here first. The flat was supposed to be ready by Easter 1985. It got to Easter and, no – the wiring hadn't been done. It went on and on like that, month after month. They kept giving us dates, then we'd come and check the place and find it wasn't ready.

It got so bad we were cracking up. We had to do everything in our power to get the work done. We got our doctors to write letters; we told our MPs; we threatened to come in here and squat. I think in the end someone realized it had gone too far and we were given another final date of 24 August 1985.

We came up and saw the architect, who said he'd put ten men on it for the last week, and he did. We found five workmen in one room doing painting jobs and five in another doing carpentry jobs! That was it. We signed the tenancy agreement and a week later we moved in.

There were still a lot of things wrong with the flat, but we were willing to accept them. The gas was off, we had no fridge, no carpet, hardly any furniture and no money at all.

# The Cost of Independence

**Kata**   It's a lot more expensive to live here than we ever imagined. We have to have central heating and it costs a fortune. That was the biggest shock – when the gas bill came. Another thing is that we can't cope with heavy amounts of cooking because it's very tiring. We use a lot of convenience foods – stuff-it-in-the-oven-jobs – and they are expensive to buy.

**Kay**   I had this wild dream that we'd be going out every night. It's not like that at all. Even if we had the money, we haven't got the energy.

**Kata**   We do go out more than we used to, and it's not such a palaver as it was when we lived with our parents, but it's not nearly on the scale we imagined.

**Kay**   We have a home help who comes in three times a week. She has her different jobs to do here and one day a week she does our food shopping. For other things, like clothes and personal shopping, we rely on friends to push us.

**Kata**   I only like my boyfriend to push me now, especially with the pavements like they are round here.

## Writing – and the Novel

**Kata**   I had a thing about writing when I was a child. Everyone else thought I was mad but I carried on, obstinately scribbling away. I never dreamt I'd meet anyone who would be remotely interested in what I was doing – and then Kay came along.

We were in hospital and I had just been ticked off by our doctor, who said, 'I look at the world today, and I can't see you earning a living by writing.' That was news to me, because I hadn't expected to earn a living by it. Anyway, there I was being told to give it all up, this writing nonsense. Kay overheard this, and it caught her interest.

**Kay**   I had been doing the same: sitting at home, writing for years, getting it all rejected and not knowing anyone. Then we got together and it was an inspiration for both of us.

**Kata**   We proceeded to write an incredibly convoluted and long novel together. It took us two years to do it. This was while we were living apart and we worked out a method of each writing the chapters. If we didn't know something, we made it up – no such thing as research for us!

**Kay**   We were only nineteen but we thought we could take on Jackie Collins. It had everything in it, this novel. We thought it was really daring. There was politics in it as well. And spying.

**Kata**   Reading it now is funny because we can see how naive we were about subjects that we know something about now, like the music business. We used to make all that up. But it was a lot of fun to do and we are rather fond of it.

A friend of mine knew an editor and the publishers saw it. They said the trouble with it was – and I think I'd agree now – that a lot of it was too sloppily written. We tended to get carried away, and in our enthusiasm we didn't bother about the writing; we just threw all our ideas down on the page.

**Kay** They didn't say throw it in the bin, but we know we'd really have to work on it to get anywhere. I couldn't face that, not now.

**Kata** It would be impossible anyway. We have just had all our stuff for the Open University course we're taking. We put ourselves down for Art and Literature and they have just sent us the lead-in work for the foundation course. I'm looking forward to that.

# Then the Band, Then the Record

**Kata** In 1981 or 1982, when we'd done the novel, I bought a keyboard. I have always liked music and singing. Ages before I met Kay, when I was at boarding school, I bullied the teachers into giving me piano lessons. I wasn't supposed to have them but I was so insistent that I ended up having lessons in the teacher's lunch-break. I only did a term, because unfortunately my fingers got too stiff and I had to give it up; but it gave me just enough knowledge to carry on later. I can't read music really, but I can do things by ear.

I played the keyboard for a bit, then I started to write songs. And we formed a band. We got some others in for this and we called ourselves 'The Decadents', much to our present embarrassment. It was another of those things we plunged into. There was a recording studio at a youth centre in Uxbridge which was quite cheap. We got in there, spent all our money and put four or five songs on cassette.

**Kay** We had our own way of doing it. We could never meet up for anything as luxurious as a rehearsal. We had one or two attempts at my house, but there was such a lot of noise and interruptions from the family.

**Kata** That was the nearest we got to rehearsing. The rest of the time I used to send Kay a tape of a song for her to learn. With the tape I'd write down the notes I wanted her to play. Fortunately, it seemed to work quite well because we all knew what we were doing when we got in the studio.

We had been doing it for fun up till then, but we thought we'd try and take it a bit further. We were completely naive: we sent the actual master tapes off to record companies, thinking they would send them back – but they never do.

Then the flat came along. The struggle to get the flat took over our lives and we had to shelve everything else, but when we got settled in here, I carried on writing songs. Some of these didn't fit in with the band so now I've gone solo and music has become the big thing for me.

Since we moved here I've had complete freedom and I've been able to get things done. I've just recorded my first single, so keep your fingers crossed for it. It's called *Live Your Life*. We decided to record it here in the flat, hiring the best-quality equipment we could get. We worked on it from ten in the morning until ten or eleven at night. We're so pleased with the way it's come out. It doesn't sound like anyone else. It's come out really well, really professional.

The other thing that's happened to me is that I've got a manager now. He looks after everything for me, which is a great help. He knows all the people we are dealing with, who are mainly from the punk scene, and he knows who is going to rip you off and who isn't. He's got a lot of sus, I would say.

When we made the first recordings with the band, which didn't get anywhere, we thought we were no good. Since then, though, other people have heard what we did and have told us we were a lot better than we thought. Now a bloke from a local record label wants to put those early songs out after the single. It's quite satisfying that there is all this interest, and that people like us.

We could still have trouble with the record companies. It's been a right year. You get the feeling there are some who just want to exploit you because you are in a wheelchair. Others say to Andy, my manager, when he goes round there, 'What does she look like?' To me that's the wrong question. I should be able to wear a paper bag over my head if I want to. I want them to say, 'What does she sound like?'

Then they might say, 'Does she do gigs?' Obviously that would be difficult for me, because of the arthritis, although I wouldn't mind performing live. I've had enough trouble lately just with studios – I can hardly get into any of them because they have steps. I don't really want to go through the effort of having someone lift me up ten flights of steps just before I have to do my big performance.

# The Fanzine

**Kata**   A lot of things have been happening lately. Someone from *Woman's Own* came down here to interview us for the magazine. They didn't put us in though. It was annoying, but we were relegated in preference to an article on Joan Collins's underwear. People from the radio are coming soon as well, and the local newspaper has already been. And between all that Kay has done her fanzine.

**Kay**   While she's been pottering around – working hard, I should say! – with her music, I've been putting together this fanzine, which is a kind of personal magazine. I've got it completed now, and it's sitting here waiting for me to get some finance so I can have it printed. It's called *Pinch Me in the Pantry*. It's got all sorts of articles in it by other people, including fan pieces on bands like The Smiths and Mark Almond. The star contributor is George Melly. We went to see him last November and I gave him a questionnaire which he sent back with his answers.

The fanzine's got a lot of art in it, as well. Really pretentious! Most fanzines look down on art, but we've got stuff on D. H. Lawrence, and poetry.

It's also got other things in it about what we call 'cripple-ism'. This is something we feel quite strongly about. Whenever we go out to a concert or a gig, the only people there in wheelchairs are me and Kata. It's true we don't go to a lot of big venues where there may be better facilities – you may get a few disabled kids going to Wembley Arena, for example – but at the places we go to, there's never anybody else in a wheelchair.

Nine times out of ten there are no facilities either. You can't get into the toilets. You've got to be carried up stairs. You've got to make all the effort. When you get in there you might be pushed into a not very good position so you're lucky if you can see anything.

**Kata**   People just don't think. Once you point things out to them, they can see what you mean. But there are still a lot of places we can't even get into. They say to us: 'You're a fire risk. You can't come in.' If you can't get in and out of the theatre by yourself, they call you a fire risk.

**Kay**   We feel we should be allowed to take the decision about whether we want to risk being burned to the ground or not. Other places can be really nice to you, but they still haven't got the facilities. Once I went to the ICA (Institute of Contemporary Art). When I got in, it was packed wall to wall: people were standing up and I couldn't see anything. So they carried me up some stairs and let me sit next to the mixing desk, where I had a really good view. But afterwards when I wanted to go to the loo the wheelchair wouldn't go through the door.

**Kata**   Half the trouble is that some places assume you aren't going to be there. It doesn't enter their heads to expect you, so they haven't got any facilities. Still ... we keep on at them.

# BUT CAN I GET IN?

The shortage of buildings with proper access and facilities for the disabled is not limited to places of entertainment, as Kay and Kata will tell you. It extends to shops, public conveniences, streets, offices and all kinds of other places.

To help you plan journeys and learn more about the facilities in particular towns and districts, RADAR (Royal Association for Disability and Rehabilitation) publishes or distributes a number of useful guides. They have a series of local access guides, of which forty to fifty are usually in print at any one time, and other titles such as *Access in the High Street* and *Access to Public Conveniences*. For information about these and other publications, contact: RADAR, Royal Association for Disability and Rehabilitation, 25 Mortimer Street, London W1N 8AB; tel. 01-637 5400.

# AT WORK

## INTRODUCTION

Sitting-down jobs are undoubtedly best for most people with arthritis. Standing-up or physical jobs, whether serving in a shop or working underground in a mine, can soon become a daily torture. In this section the contributors describe how they came to terms with their limitations.

Adaptation need not involve a change of career, though this may be necessary. The first aim is usually to find a way of modifying the working method. Most people succeed, but it can be a daunting struggle to find the motivation from day to day.

Meanwhile there are other options to full-time work: a part-time job, perhaps, or work that can be done from home on a more casual basis. The youngest of these contributors, Judith Fitzgerald, is convinced that people of her generation should make it their priority to get the best possible qualifications they can, through education, before seeking a way into the jobs market.

# THE SPORTSMAN

## David Icke

At the age of fifteen David Icke looked forward to a full career in professional football. Then he developed arthritis and at twenty-one had to give up the game. Here he tells the story of what happened and how he switched to journalism, working his way up to become a sports presenter on BBC television.

About six months after I joined Coventry City Football Club my left knee swelled up, for no apparent reason. There was no pain, but the swelling did not go down. I had various tests, which were all negative, and was told, 'We can't explain it. So play on.'

I did, but over the next few years the arthritis began to spread. I got a swollen right ankle which, unlike the knee, was very painful. Then it went into my right knee and my career was finished. Thirteen years ago I came out of professional football and since then the arthritis has gone into some of my fingers, both wrists and both ankles; my toes are bad as well.

At the time it was first diagnosed as arthritis, it was always called rheumatoid arthritis. A few years ago I went to see my local doctor for an insurance medical. I told him my story, and he put me on to a guy who had just joined his practice who had been studying arthritis. He examined my joints and fingers and said I had classic symptoms of psoriatic arthritis. So that is what he and I now believe it is. Whatever you call it, though, doesn't make it less painful.

I had joined Coventry City straight from school, and at first I tried to put up with the pain and get on with the only career I had known, the only thing I ever wanted to do. By the time I was nineteen the pain was very bad and I had to accept, hard though it was, that I would not be able to continue.

I had already agreed as much with the Coventry club when a famous old player called John Charles stepped in. He was managing a non-League team, Hereford United, and he rang me

103

and asked if I fancied joining them. At that time Hereford trained two evenings a week and played on Saturdays or midweek. That sounded easier than what I had been doing and, as I had no other prospects, I decided to give it a try.

During the next two years I went through agony. The twenty-minute warm-ups before training – when all the joints were cold – were the worst times. On match days the adrenaline was there and I could cope better.

The club, meanwhile, was doing really well and was elected to the Football League. I played in goal for Hereford during their first season in the League. I had sixty games. The first forty-odd were painful, and the training was terrible to endure. Then, probably because the team was doing well and heading for promotion, I somehow found the pain was disappearing, even though the swelling remained. I thought I had cracked it; but I was wrong.

At the end of the season I went on the club's tour to Spain, organized as a kind of celebration. Less than a week after we were back, I woke up one morning and could not move anything. I was finished as a footballer, and never played again.

It was small consolation at the time, but at least my problems were fully out in the open. I would no longer have to pretend I had something else wrong with me as a way of disguising the truth. The club knew something of my troubles, but if I had told them the whole story they would have lost confidence in me. So on one morning I would complain of blisters which were not really there. Another day I'd say, 'Got this kick yesterday; I'm a bit sore this morning.' They thought I was a hypochondriac. It became a standing joke: 'What's wrong with Ickey today?' Now, however, the problem was clear for all to see. For three or four days my wife had to just about carry me around the house. After two weeks the club cancelled my contract. I was out, landed in that frightening position where money was going out but not a penny was coming in, and with no sign of a career.

## A New Start

I decided I wanted to become a television sports presenter with the BBC. A lot of people found that extremely funny. An out-of-work professional footballer who at times could hardly walk, and who had never passed an exam in his life – what use was he to anyone, let alone the BBC?

As a first step into journalism, and after a lot of refusals, I got a job on a weekly paper in Leicester. I sold the house in Hereford (just in time) and went from being a £100-a-week footballer to a £23-a-week news reporter.

I stayed six months in Leicester, then worked my way up through a news agency, then an evening paper, followed by local radio, and finally I got into the BBC. Once you have got your first job in journalism, nobody bothers about your lack of qualifications: you're in. As I went on, I felt enormous determination to overcome the adversity of arthritis and what it had done to my life, and this must have helped me to fight my way to where I wanted to be.

As much as I can, I try to treat the arthritis with contempt. I force myself to do things. Once you give in to it on any regular basis – there are times you *have* to give in because it's unbearable otherwise – you soon find yourself going backwards.

The pain goes in phases. It grew worse after I stopped playing football and I have always had to struggle with it. A few months ago I had a bad patch, but since then I have been on a new diet which has been tremendously helpful. My wrist is still painful, but I have not felt so well in myself for a very long time.

As for my work, the quality of what I do, I am better off than I was before. When I was playing football I enjoyed the matches – it was fantastic playing in front of a crowd – but a lot of the in-between stuff was frankly quite boring. I don't miss that at all. My life is now much richer and more full as a result of no longer being a professional footballer. In that negative sense my arthritis has done me a favour. It forced me to look again at my life and find a new challenge. For five years it was very hard work while I learned my new career and tried to catch up with my contemporaries. Fortunately, I have a competitive nature; I took my opportunities and kept going.

Always there has been the arthritis, but I have refused to let it dominate my life. Until the day they carry me out, I will go on fighting it.

# THE MP

## Jo Richardson

Jo Richardson, MP, has had rheumatoid arthritis for nearly thirty years. The onset of the disease did not prevent her from pursuing her career in politics and she continues to fulful a busy schedule with a special interest in women's matters. She lives by herself in a flat in London.

It came on quite suddenly. My knee swelled up and I started to limp. I didn't know what it was. I was not then an MP but I was working for someone who was, Barnett Stross. Eventually he said to me, 'I think you've got arthritis.' I told him not to be ridiculous, but he insisted I saw a consultant, who confirmed that it was rheumatoid arthritis. Over the years it showed in my hands and began to crop up all over me. I would wake up one morning and it would be in the back of my neck or in my shoulders; then it would appear somewhere else.

At the hospital I dealt with a series of registrars, some of whom I liked and some I did not. The strangest of them told me I would only get better if I turned to God – hardly my idea of professional advice. In fact, I couldn't believe what I was hearing. In the middle of a busy outpatients' clinic he explained that none of the things I was taking would do me any good; my only hope was to turn to God. I didn't go back there for some time.

I then changed to my present consultant and everything is very much better. He is enthusiastic and good at explaining things – not one of those people who treat you over the top of your head, as if you weren't there.

I have tried all kinds of treatments since I first got arthritis. In the sixties I tried acupuncture, but I had to give it up after one visit because I couldn't afford the fees. They wanted £7 a time, which in those days was nearly as much as my salary, and I was meant to go once a week. People still come up to me and recommend these herbal baths and those thermal baths and so on, and sometimes I try them. They may give me some temporary relief, but that is all; so mostly I don't bother.

I was treated with cortisone for some time, but then it was decided to take me off it, which took two years. I also took some paracetamol, but then, to compensate for the lack of cortisone, I started – on my own – to take more paracetamol. I found it helped, whereas other drugs I was being prescribed only made me feel ill. In the end I threw the others away, except for one which I use occasionally to reduce inflammation. I work on the theory that if I am stiff painkillers will kill the pain and allow me to move again. So I take six paracetamol whenever I feel stiffness coming on. My consultant isn't keen on my taking such a quantity, but he accepts that it works for me.

A few years ago we did an experiment. During a parliamentary recess, I agreed not to take any paracetamol for a week. I said that paracetamol kept the swelling down; my consultant said that it couldn't. He gave me a measure so that I could keep a chart monitoring the swelling on my fingers. During the week they got puffier and puffier and bigger and bigger. I showed him the chart at the end of the week and he took it and waved it at his colleagues. 'My patient is proving us all wrong,' he said.

So I stick to paracetamol and I get by. I don't expect to get rid of the arthritis; the bones are too set. I go to the hospital every three months for another prescription. My worst problem is my feet. My hands are bent, but I can manage to write and type; lifting things is difficult, so usually I get someone else to do that.

My ankles are weak and this affects my balance. I have a private horror of going to a meeting hall and having to climb the four or five steps to the platform with no rail to help me. To do it by myself is petrifying. I usually ask someone if I can hang on to their arm. It's a curious fear, because if there *is* a rail I can go up and down the steps without touching it.

I try to avoid stairs, where possible. The House of Commons is not an ideal place for anyone to work, let alone someone with arthritis, but at least there are lifts. To reach one you may have to walk down a long corridor, but you can get from one level to another without using the stairs.

I have given up going on demonstrations or marches. Now I go straight to the destination and meet the marchers as they come in. The last march I went on was about three years ago, for CND.

It nearly killed me. I started at the front and finished at the back. I would have dropped out, but there was nowhere to drop out *to*. All the buses had been diverted, there were no taxis; there was nowhere to go but on. I know I shouldn't have tried to do the march; I won't make that mistake again.

# Getting About

I have a car and when I am in London I use it as much as possible. A car is much handier than public transport for getting round a constituency and making calls. I am glad I do not have to depend on public transport in London; I have a lot of sympathy for disabled people who have to struggle on and off buses, and who can't get down the aisle with their sticks because it isn't wide enough. I find the underground easier to manage, although stairs are always a problem. Trains, especially the InterCity 125s, are difficult to get in and out of: the step is too narrow and, when leaving the train, I have to put one foot sideways onto the step, then bring my other foot level with it, then reach down for the platform. Not easy.

My constituents know about my arthritis and they have always been sympathetic. Nobody has ever said, 'You shouldn't be doing this.' They just pile more work on me. Perhaps some people find it easier to relate to me because I have a disability. 'You've got your problems,' they say, then pour out their own.

My friends in the House of Commons give me help and support. They will pick up a bag for me without being asked, that kind of thing. There is one set of interview rooms in the House which has very difficult door handles: you have to twist them. I can't manage that so I have to ask someone to do it for me. That is all right if I am having a meeting with people who know me, but with strangers it can be awkward. There I am, conducting a meeting, giving orders – 'We're going to do this, we're going to do that' – then at the end of it I can't even open the door!

I am lucky in that I can do my job without any special difficulty. I have to walk about a bit, but I am able to do that. I can stand for about an hour if I have to, and the rest of the time I can spend sitting down. It must be terrible if you need to use your limbs as an essential part of your job. If I had been working in a shop, for instance, when I first got arthritis, I would not have been able to carry on.

# THE LOCAL
# GOVERNMENT
# OFFICER

## Peter Nightingale

Peter Nightingale has had rheumatoid arthritis since he was
eight. He has had two hip and two knee replacement operations. He is also a diabetic. He left school after taking A levels
and in 1973 entered local government. Recently he passed
the Diploma of Management Studies.

The arthritis is quite good at the moment. My left ankle gets
very painful if I stand up too long, my right knee is going through
a bad phase, and my neck is very stiff, but it varies all the time;
it is never consistent. Some people get arthritis in one place –
say, the right arm – and that's it. I've got it generally all over,
and the pain comes through in different places.

I have trouble raising my arms, but I have grown used to that.
I look on the arthritis as something that happened a long time
ago which has left me with a certain amount of limited
movement. To me it is normal to be like I am. That doesn't mean
it's not painful, but I have learnt to do things by moving the non-
painful bits if I can.

At school I was lucky and did not lose a lot of time through ill-
health – about one month a year on average, when I was in
hospital. When I was eleven I passed the exam to go to a
grammar school, but it could not cope with me and I had to go to
a handicapped school for a year. Apart from that I managed
school OK, and finished with quite good results. I did A levels,
left school when I was eighteen, immediately went into hospital
for seven months, then came out and got a job. That was in April
1973 and I've been working ever since. If it had been a few years

later, with the recession starting, it would have been much more difficult, but when I was looking there were jobs available.

When I was very young I'd had bigger ambitions, but after school I was basically looking for some sort of job. I started in a local government office and now I work at Hammersmith Town Hall in West London where I have the very grand title of Office Services Manager. This means I am responsible for the office and particularly the filing or information system, which has a small library attached to it.

To help me at work I have a high-seat chair, which is easier to get in and out of. I am left-handed, which meant I used to have a problem with telephoning as I cannot get my right hand up to my head. I got round this by devising a special aid – a long handle which grips the receiver and holds it at head level while I hold the other end with my right hand down at desk level.

At home I have an aid for putting on socks and shoes. I can also attach a brush to it to comb the back of my head; I couldn't reach otherwise. I can't manage ties and I can't do the top buttons on my shirt – I can get only about halfway up. Dressing takes time. I get up at six-thirty and allow an hour for it. It's one of those things. A fellow in my section gets up at eight and he's in the office by nine. I can't do that.

As for the future: my office and others like it must eventually move away from their old-fashioned manual systems and become computerized. That will be something for me to get involved in, but I also hope that in time I will be able to shift into a more broad-based management career, concerned with planning and decision-making. I have already participated in a number of working parties – partly, but not wholly, because I have special knowledge of what it's like to be disabled. These working parties have been largely concerned with how local authorities see themselves consulting and serving the public.

At one time I was a shop steward, and then after two years of that I switched into doing voluntary work for Arthritis Care. I have always liked to keep the two things – main job and voluntary work – running side by side. Up until now my job has been fairly routine and I have been glad of the opportunity to do something slightly more challenging in my spare time. Now the experience I have acquired doing voluntary work looks as if it will help me take on bigger assignments in my full-time career.

# THE JOURNALIST

## Marje Proops

Marje Proops of the *Daily Mirror* is one of Britain's best-loved and most celebrated columnists, but she nearly had to pack it all in when arthritis attacked her in both hips and soon left her confined to a wheelchair. For five years she fought the disease, but then she had two hip replacement operations and came safely through. Now she is back on her feet again – and still working at the desk she never really left.

I first began to realize that something funny was going on about twenty years ago. It started with back problems. I thought it was straightforward disc trouble, and so did the doctors. One day when it was very bad, I was seeing a consultant. He said, 'You've got a back like a row of beads. I'm afraid you have arthritis.'

I said, 'What's arthritis?'

I didn't know what it was or what it meant. I knew nothing whatsoever about it. Gradually, of course, I learnt about it, and I discovered that what it meant was agonizing pain.

The arthritis settled, not in the spine where it first showed itself, but in the hips. As the weeks went by, they grew more and more painful, and I became less and less mobile. I went to see another specialist, who confirmed what was wrong with me. In due course, he said, I would have to have hip replacements. But not yet: I wasn't sufficiently advanced in age and the arthritis wasn't 'ripe' enough to operate.

By that time I was walking with the aid of two sticks. Then I had to use crutches. During all this time I was having physiotherapy at the local hospital to try to keep the mobility going and to ease the pain a bit. I was taking pills and painkillers, but the disease marched on despite anything that anybody tried to do.

One day in my office I stood up from my desk to walk across the room. Nothing happened. My legs simply refused to obey their usual instruction to 'go'.

It frightened me. I sat down again and rang up the newspaper's Medical Department.

'I can't walk!' I told them.

They sent me a wheelchair, accompanied by a nurse who helped me into it. As soon as I was settled I rang my orthopaedic consultant, only to find he was away on holiday.

'You'll have to stay in that wheelchair until he comes back,' his receptionist told me, 'and then we'll see.'

So there I was. Stuck in a wheelchair for the first time in my life, and having to face the fact that I was badly disabled.

I was to be condemned to a wheelchair for five and a half years. I returned the borrowed one and got my own, but right from the start I was determined not to let it ruin my life.

I went to my office every day. I told myself that I was still functioning perfectly well from the hips upwards, and if, so far as I knew, there was nothing wrong with my head, I could still get on with my work. So I did.

I will not pretend there were not problems. There were severe problems. But despite all the limiting factors I was able to develop a routine. Each morning I was driven to the office, loaded into my wheelchair and pushed to the lift. At the front door they telephoned my secretary and she met me at the lift and wheeled me to my office, where I sat and worked at my desk as I always had done.

## Helpful People

I was certainly lucky in that I was never left to cope in isolation, as some people are. I was always surrounded by helpful people who would push me wherever I needed to go. Twice a day I attend an editorial conference in the Editor's office, which is at the far end of the building from my office. Somebody was always available to wheel me there. In fact, they used to time it. They had competitions to see who could get me to the Editor's office in the quickest time! The Picture Editor always won: he was the only one allowed to take the short cut through the Dark Room. They were all very competitive and I had to cling on to the arms of the wheelchair like anything while they swung me round corners. One enthusiast even managed to tip me out!

I thought I would be more independent if I got myself an electric wheelchair, so I wouldn't need to have someone pushing me everywhere. Unfortunately, the carpets in the corridors were joined in those days by narrow metal strips which formed little ridges on the surface – and the electric wheelchair used to get stuck on these.

On one horrendous occasion I got myself trapped in a ladies' loo on the ninth floor. I had driven myself along there, all independent, and not until I was stuck inside did I come to appreciate one important thing about that particular loo: hardly anyone else ever used it. Before someone at last released me, I was a helpless prisoner for quite some time. It wasn't a huge drama, but it's the sort of thing you don't forget.

In my time I endured many of the things that the wheelchair-bound learn to put up with. A lot of people – by which I mean able-bodied people – somehow get it into their heads that you-down-there are different. So they carry on conversations over the top of you. They say to the person pushing you, 'How is she today?', as if you're deaf or don't speak the language. 'Is she feeling better?' they go on. 'Is she in pain?'

After the first few times, I grew accustomed to it, even amused by it. I certainly didn't let it upset me. There are compensations, too, if you have to spend your days sitting chest-high to everyone else – everyone, that is, except children. Children don't see you as a disabled person. You are on the same eye level as they are, and so they come bounding up and talk to you. I had a lot of great conversations with kids – and with dogs as well, except for the ones which lifted their leg on the wheelchair.

Perhaps I should except my colleagues at work from what I have just said about the able-bodied and their attitudes. My colleagues gave me wonderful support and they did it in a jokey, understanding way. They called me 'Old Mother Ironside' and shouted things like, 'Out of the way! Here comes our favourite cripple!'

They had the sense not to pretend that I was able-bodied, and I was grateful for it. Their good-natured jokes made it much easier for me to cope with my troubles. In circumstances like mine, the worst thing anyone could have said was, 'Oh, you poor dear' and 'How awful for you'. I would have hated any of that.

You never completely adjust to your lack of mobility. In the office, for example, I could not reach all my books and if I wanted one from an upper shelf I had to ask my secretary to come in and get it down for me. To someone who is not used to being waited on hand and foot, this is irritating, but you have to face the fact that there are things you simply cannot do without the help of others. For the rest, I concentrated on getting on with my life and with my work.

My worst travelling experience came about when I had to go to the Albert Hall to judge a competition. I rang them up in advance to ask if they had a wheelchair I could use, or if I should bring my own. No, no, they assured me, they would provide a wheelchair and someone to look after me and wheel me wherever I had to go. Fine, I thought, I don't have to worry about that any more.

When I arrived, however, there were blank faces all round. No-one knew anything about it. There was no wheelchair, and I had just sent mine away in the boot of the car. I was completely stuck. The next bit of bad news was that the judging was taking place on a lower floor; there was no lift, only stairs. There was nothing for it. I went down those stairs on my bottom – hardly the sort of entrance for a judge to make! Or anyone else for that matter.

# Liberty at Last

I would have had my first hip replacement done sooner, but I had to wait because in the meantime something else went wrong with me. I had a blocked carotid artery, and while this was being investigated under anaesthetic, I sustained a small stroke. This led to some paralysis down one arm and in three fingers, and I had to wait a year while this sorted itself out – which it eventually did – before the great day came for the hip operation.

I had wanted both hips done together, but the specialist disagreed. The operation was a success and I emerged from it halfway on the road to recovery, though now with one leg slightly shorter than the other, which meant I had to wear a specially built-up shoe for a year. However, the surgeon promised faithfully that when I had the second operation he would make my other leg exactly the same length as the first. He was as good as his word.

And here I am. I have two tin hips, or whatever they're made of. I can walk, dance, run, do nearly anything short of active sports. I can't walk very far, but I can go a short distance – a hundred yards or so – as fast as I want; then I stop for a rest until the ache goes away, and carry on.

I feel a certain amount of fatigue, but that may be from my age as much as from the arthritis. It's difficult to tell. I try to compare myself with my sister, who is about eighteen months younger than I am, and apart from the distance walking, I can do just as much as she can.

Looking back over the whole experience, I am convinced that the only way to recover from any kind of severe illness is through sheer willpower: mind over matter. I was utterly determined that I wasn't going to be a cripple and that I wasn't going to have to be looked after for a minute longer than was necessary.

I really disliked the whole business of having to be bathed, dressed, and have my hair washed by someone else. I couldn't do anything for myself and was completely dependent on others – my husband mostly, and he was wonderful, but I found it awful. I had always regarded myself as an able-bodied woman, but then to have to sit there while my husband put my tights on for me – that was something I found very hard.

## Learning about Pain

I also learned a few things about pain. At work it is something you keep to yourself. With colleagues you are bound to put on a brave face. They all have their jobs to do, and you have to watch out that you don't take advantage of their kindness and goodwill. Only my husband and my son knew about the pain I suffered. Only in the intimacy of family life, with people you feel really close to, can you relax, let go, and say, 'Yes. It hurts. I'm in agony.'

And then you cry. And swear. And let your feelings go. That was a very necessary part of life for me. It must be terrible for people who don't have others they can confide in and who have to keep up an act the whole time, either because their family are impatient and reluctant to make allowances for another person's illness, or because there is no-one around.

I think, though, that the sufferer has to be careful. Pain is a very subjective matter, and difficult to measure in others. So if you do complain, perhaps you shouldn't do it too often –

especially if you look reasonably well in yourself. There must be a tendency for everyone's nearest and dearest to think, 'Why does she have to make such a bloody fuss? Does she think she's the only person in the world who's got pain in the hips (or whatever)?'

No, taking advantage of one's nearest and dearest is not a good idea. Nor is it a good idea to let yourself become too self-centred about your pain. From there it would be only too easy to slide into a self-pitying attitude and you would soon end up wondering where all your friends had gone.

In my own case, I have to remember at all times that I have been lucky. I do get swellings and some pain in my fingers, which is worse when the weather is hot and dry; but my main problem, with the hips, has been dealt with and I can regard it as a closed episode. As I said to the surgeon before my first operation, 'I'm glad I'm not my cat. At least I've only got two hips!'

# THE MUSICIAN

## Michael Morrow

---

Michael Morrow suffers from haemarthrosis. This stems from his having Christmas Disease, in which a coagulation factor in the blood, known as Factor 9, is missing. He became an expert in medieval Renaissance music and his group, Musica Reservata, is one of the best-known in this field. Recently, however, he has found it difficult to continue.

---

As a child I had bruised joints a lot and the only thing one could do in those days was to stay in bed until they got better. After the war treatment improved a bit, with blood transfusions being more readily given. I was able to live a reasonably normal life until, some while ago now, I broke my leg.

Since then, having had a spell in hospital, all these problems from my childhood have caught up with me in the form of arthritis. For instance, on a number of occasions I have slipped, as anyone might, and put my hand out to break the fall; but because of the arthritis I have not been able to put my arm out straight and so it has simply broken above the elbow, the weakest place. As a result I am now terrified of falling.

The arthritis, which arises from blood leaking into joints and destroying them, affects me most in the knees, elbows and ankles; the back of my neck isn't too good either. At one time I badly needed an operation on my right hip; I could hardly sit in a chair. Due to a marvellous concentrate of Factor 9 which now exists, the doctors can make my blood almost normal, and because of this I have been able to have the hip replaced. I am not, however, as mobile as I would wish to be, and do not go out much.

All this history of operations, hospitals and problems with my blood has brought me over the years to a position where I find it almost impossible to work. At the hospital they say I am going through a depression; it's something they are trying to find out about. I want to work more than anything. In the beginning I did a bit of teaching, and since then have spent the last twenty-five years transcribing and performing medieval Renaissance music. I used to play the lute and various wind instruments, which I cannot do at present since breaking my arm a couple of times. In my work, though, I have been less concerned with playing myself than with finding other very good people to play and directing them.

The group is called Musica Reservata. We held a lot of concerts at London's Queen Elizabeth Hall and elsewhere, and made a number of gramophone records. The group's name is a bit of a joke. It is a term found in sixteenth-century music but, as yet, nobody knows what it means. I was recently told off by a German lady who wanted me to be moderator at a harp symposium. She was appalled that a group could be so lightly named. 'You muss be serious about ziss sings,' was her attitude; but it is part of me that I do not behave in a serious way about things which actually concern me. Since there is so much that is not known – in fact, what one does know is hardly the tip of the iceberg – I think Musica Reservata is rather a good name. Suitably pompous as well!

Recently, though, the mental strain of working, of preparing for concerts, has been too much for me. By the time we reach the first rehearsal and everyone has their music, I can relax and begin to enjoy myself. It's the part before that which is so difficult, when I have to choose or transcribe the music. At present I get a form of mental seizure which prevents me from even starting.

I am having physiotherapy to strengthen my muscles, which I think is marvellous, but at the moment I suffer from awful periods of lethargy. I can rise out of it, if someone telephones or comes to see me and we find something interesting to say to each other, but when they are gone I quickly sink back into it.

There are projects lined up, waiting for me to do. I am supposed to produce an edition of some dances from the mid-sixteenth century which are *terribly* corrupt in the printed source. They are four-, five- and six-part dances, and are more or less self-contained single manuscripts. The great problem is that the cantus part, which in most cases contains the tune, is missing from the collection. It's a job, really, without an end.

There are so many mistakes in the manuscripts, which are mainly collected from other printed sources, that they are totally unplayable as they stand – though I know they have been used to play from.

The book has three hundred and twenty-two pieces in it, and there is a second book which I am trying not to think about! I have done a lot of the work. I have got together about thirty-odd out of the sixty-odd six-part pieces, and all I need to do is check a few things, write something about it – and it's done. But I can't do it.

At the hospital they sent me to see a psychiatrist. He is a very pleasant chap and tells me about where he is going on holiday; but it seems to me quite pointless.

The thing with me is, I don't expect miracles, but I always feel there is a possibility of one. If only there could be a way of getting to that state.

I always used to work day and night. My wife used to complain about it! She now says she wishes those days were back.

I would like to discuss this with other haemophiliacs, because they will know the kind of thing I am going through. It must be rather like what is called writer's block, something you have to force yourself out of. I just wish there was a way I could get about more, walk up and down the road and go to the shops, for example; but with the arthritis I can't get that far. I don't know.

# THE NOVELIST

## Rosemary Sutcliff

Rosemary Sutcliff is a popular and much-praised writer. She contracted Still's Disease as a child, and in *Blue Remembered Hills* she recalls her life and its physical and emotional trials up to the time her first book was accepted for publication. She has now written more than forty novels. She lives and works in her house in West Sussex.

I can walk around with the help of elbow-crutches, and I have a wheelchair for out-of-doors. I need help with getting up in the morning and going to bed at night, but otherwise I am fairly self-sufficient.

I have two people to help me run the house: a housekeeper who lives in, and a gardener who lives in a cottage by the gate. He drives the car and comes to the rescue when fuses blow, and so on.

I have always tried to live as independently as possible. When my mother was alive, she looked after me in our house in Devon. She was always saying that she felt terrible about leaving me; what would happen to me after she had gone, she wanted to know. I knew that I would be fine, but I couldn't tell her that, which was sad.

After she died, I moved up to this house in West Sussex with my father. I was an up-and-coming writer and we decided it would be better to be closer to the publishers. My father lived here for eleven years before he died, and I have been paddling my own canoe ever since.

## The Working Day

I begin the day with breakfast in bed. I am up by about half-past eight, or a quarter to nine, then I finish getting washed and dressed and go into the room where I work. My two chihuahuas follow me around, and I can usually see some doves on the lawn outside – there is a dovecote in the garden.

The next thing I do is to spend quite a long time hovering around, either reading the newspaper or doing whatever I can in a standing position. The reason for this is that my bottom gives out if I sit on it too early in the day and then try to do a lot of work. One of the sitting bones gets very sore, especially when I have lost a bit of weight – which I can do at the drop of a hat. I can always lose weight, but I can't put it on again.

About mid-morning I sit down and start work. Then for the rest of the day I work, off and on, reserving to myself the right to stop and go out for the afternoon if I want to, or to take time off if friends drop in. This is the thing for me: I reckon on doing piecework rather than completing a fixed number of hours.

No-one respects the hours of a woman writer working at home, and friends do sometimes drop in at frustrating moments when I am in the middle of an important piece or the fluency is going really well. I long ago gave up trying to do so-many hours in a day; now I try to get so-much work done instead. If necessary I carry on working later, or start earlier, or take work to bed with me. Quite often I don't get as much piecework finished as I might have hoped to, but if I have written a thousand words I reckon that's been a good day.

I write my books in longhand and am lucky that I enjoy doing it this way. If I had to use a dictaphone or something like that, I would find it much more difficult. I usually write three drafts, all the way through, and then the final one goes off to be turned into a typescript for the publishers. They, of course, won't touch anything that is handwritten.

I was twenty-eight when my first book came out, and I have now written, I think, forty-five, counting the short ones for children's series, which works out at a bit more than a book a year. The book I am working on now is for adults. I have been writing it for two years so far, and it will probably take another eight months to finish.

This story has been a brute to write because it is set in unfamiliar countries – Egypt and Arabia – and takes place, to make matters slightly more involved, in the early nineteenth century, from 1804 to 1814. It has taken me a long time to do the research, having to stop and think about things which I would have known immediately if I had been writing about, say, Roman Britain. I belong to the County Library and the London Library, and by following up 'Further Reading' lists and other references I can usually, by a snowballing process, build up a picture of the place I want to describe. This present book has been more difficult because not much has been written on the subject. A little while ago I wrote to Kew Gardens in despair to ask them about the flowers of the Western Desert. They wrote back saying, 'Terribly sorry, you've hit on our one completely blank spot. There is no book about the flowers of the Western Desert, though one is due to come out in five years' time.' That is the kind of thing that has slowed me up.

I used to go on marvellous trips abroad, to Greece and other places, but the people I went with aren't around now. I *would* still go on a big journey if the right chance arose. I don't mind any form of transport, except planes. I have flown several times but I really can't stand it. I feel physically ill, claustrophobic, agoraphobic, disorientated – you name it, I feel it. It's got nothing to do with being disabled – in fact, it's a nuisance because flying would be much the simplest way for me to travel a long distance.

## A Fountain Pen and a Bottle of Ink

I look upon myself as a full-time working girl. I left school at fourteen and went to art school. I was virtually uneducable at that time, and have picked up all my education since, teaching myself. I did a three-year course at art school, by which time the war had begun, and then I started to paint miniatures. I hadn't really wanted to go in for miniatures, but because of my arthritis my family thought I would find big canvases too difficult to deal with. At one time I saw myself becoming the first woman President of the Royal Academy. Then gradually I discovered that writing appealed to me more, so I made the switch.

I don't think there has ever been a time, since I left school, when I didn't have some aim in view, some job that I could do. I have been very lucky with writing, because it is creative; I love doing it and am able to do it without problems.

My writing desk is my old painting desk. On it I keep various things in layers. At the bottom is my diary; next is a disreputable-looking object which is my address book; and on top is the book of the moment, a large notebook which has all my scraps of notes in it.

I have always written with a fountain pen, which I dip in the ink bottle rather than fill; one dip usually lasts for about an eighth of a page. I can't use a biro. Fountain pens are not what they used to be; the nibs are so rigid and unspringy. My first writing pen, with which I wrote several of my early books, cost me 1s 9d (about 9p). It was so lovely to have a nib that was sensitive and springy. After it broke its back I lashed it up with adhesive tape and carried on using it until, eventually, it started to suck instead of blow; sadly I accepted that it had to go.

Those few things – a desk, my notes, a book to write in, a fountain pen and a bottle of ink – are really the extent of my working equipment. Those same items have kept me in business for almost forty years. I have been lucky.

# THE TYPIST

## David Webb

David Webb has a dual disability. At the age of seven he contracted Still's Disease, which affected his eyesight as well as his joints; within three years he was totally blind. He was educated at a special school for the blind, then went to a commercial college and learnt shorthand and typing. Now thirty-five, he lives in a flat in West London, which he is buying through a housing association.

The arthritis started in my knees, then it affected my ankles, then both elbows, one wrist and some fingers in my right hand. Between 1958 and 1967, when the disease was at its most active, I was very up and down. I was laid low for long periods and virtually had to learn to walk again.

In the last few years my mobility has been quite good. Moving around my flat, or in the corridors at work, I manage pretty well. I wouldn't venture very far in the street, though: my balance is delicate and I could easily topple over on a rough pavement. When I am confident, I have quite good mobility, but confidence is easily shattered. If I am going to the local market or shops, I prefer to have a friend push me in a wheelchair.

My eyes began to trouble me before my joints. I was at a boarding school in East London at the time, and I vaguely remember being taken to what I knew then as the Marylebone Eye Hospital; now it's called the Western Ophthalmic. I spent a few days in there, went back to the school and then, a few weeks later, my knees began to hurt. The first time I realized this was when I was on shoe-cleaning duty in the dormitory; I found I was having difficulty in bending. When I looked down, I saw that one of my knees was puffed up and swollen. From then on, the problems I had with my eyes and my joints advanced together. By the age of ten I was totally blind.

I am a little bit hazy about what precisely happened. When I first got the disease I was too young to understand what was going on. Later, when I was in a position to ask for information, I'd had it so long I'd kind of lost interest. As I understand it now, the same inflammation that attacks the joints also attacks a certain part of the eye. In 1976 I had an operation to remove a cataract and they found that the inflammation had destroyed the retina. It was like removing a curtain to find that the window was sooted up.

My family then moved to Nottingham and by that Christmas I was in a children's hospital there, from which I didn't emerge for three years. My education during that time was virtually non-existent, except for what I could pick up on the BBC schools programmes. I was in the first throes of the disease and dealing with that took up most of the time anyway. I learnt braille after about eighteen months, and then I was able to do a little bit of schoolwork.

When I came out of hospital I was ten, and it was decided that I should go through the system of education for the blind. I was entered for Worcester College for the Blind, which provides a grammar school education. I did all the usual subjects – Maths, English, French, German, Latin and History – and eventually I took my O levels. After that I passed A levels in History and English.

Braille machines have progressed a lot in the last thirty years, just as typewriters have. Many years ago people learnt braille on a hand frame, painstakingly dotting out each dot one by one. By the time I was at school we had a machine called a Perkins, in which you insert a sheet of paper as you do into a typewriter and then hit the keys. There are only six keys and these punch the dots into the paper. The teachers, of course, have to know braille as well so they can follow what you are doing.

I had a number of severe flare-ups and my education had to be suspended for long periods while I was in hospital. By the time I left school I was twenty. Then I went to a commercial training college in London, run by the RNIB (Royal National Institute for the Blind), and learnt shorthand and typing.

Three weeks after leaving college I got myself a job and, touch wood, I have been in work ever since. My first job was at the London office of an Australian firm called Burns Philp, which is a big trading company in the South Seas with department stores, garages and other interests. I was the shorthand typist to the export manager for most of my time there.

The office was in Kingsway, in central London, and to start with I lived in a hostel for the blind in Holland Park, West London. Then I moved to a place which offered semi-sheltered housing for the blind, in Goldhawk Road. Each day I went to work by minicab and came home the same way. I got an allowance towards my fare but had to find the rest myself. Around 1979, I think, there was an oil crisis and cab fares went up a lot. I was having to pay too much out of my own pocket, so I decided I'd better find another job quick.

A friend who works for the Social Services in the borough of Westminster suggested I try them. He said typing jobs in the Social Services were more interesting than most. So I applied to the boroughs of Hammersmith and Kensington & Chelsea, as they were nearer to where I was living. Both offered me an interview. The Hammersmith offices were not really suitable for me because they were reached by a very spiral staircase, but at the other place, in Ladbroke Grove, there were no problems and they offered me the job. That is where I work now. Mainly, for my sins, I take minutes at child abuse case conferences, edit them and produce a typed report for the chairman.

## Housing Problems – and a Solution

I now have my own flat, which suits me best out of all the places I have lived in. It's a lot better than the hostel, where I had very little privacy, and a good bit better than the semi-sheltered place where I lived for seven years.

Space has a lot to do with it. In the Goldhawk Road place I had my own room but shared the kitchen and bathroom. Everything in the kitchen was duplicated, and my half of the space was about 5 ft (1.5 m) long and 3 ft (1 m) wide. I had to pack all my other things into my room; in the end I had a fridge-freezer in there, and a dining table, a bed, a settee, a stereo ... I was getting seriously short of space, and also by then I was that much older and felt that I had mentally grown out of this kind of arrangement. Another point was that, as long as I went on paying rent, I was getting no investment benefit. I started looking around for somewhere to buy.

This was not easy, but I was fortunate. My problem, like most first-time buyers, was getting on the ladder. On my salary I could not borrow enough to buy a flat in the right area (the right area being anywhere within a reasonable cab-ride of Ladbroke Grove). I decided how much I could afford to spend on fares then worked out that this gave me about a 4 mile (6 km) radius from Ladbroke Grove. As property would be cheaper to the west, going out of London, I tried to find somewhere in Acton, which was about the furthest point.

There was nothing. The cost of property far exceeded what I could afford and even if I could have raised the extra, it would not have worked. The repayments would have been huge in relation to what I was earning, and the cab fares would also have been more than I really wanted to pay.

Then another possibility suddenly turned up. I go to a disabled swimming club which meets every Friday, and one night one of the lifeguards happened to mention that he was getting a place under a part-ownership scheme with a housing association. Why didn't I try that?

I didn't really know anything about housing associations, but he told me he was dealing with the Addison Housing Association, which is the selling arm of Notting Hill Housing Trust. I applied and was told that a block of flats was opening in Shepherds Bush. As I was living just down the road, they asked me to come and view it. When I arrived, there were hundreds of other people, and all I kept remembering was the bit on the form which said that priority would be given to people who were already clients of the Trust. Without much hope I said I would like one of the flats and went home. Next thing, they rang up and said, 'We can offer you Flat No. 1. If you'd like to make up your mind ....'

The deal was that I could buy the flat by taking out a mortgage on a quarter of the price and paying a reasonable rent on the rest. This is what I decided to do; alternatively, if I had wanted, I could have borrowed half the amount or three quarters. The total price was fixed by the District Valuer. It works out that my rent for three quarters is about one and a half times what I pay on the mortgage for the one quarter. I wish now I had bought a half at the beginning, because property prices have gone mad around here and when I do take on another quarter it's going to cost me a lot more. All the same, I have made a start. For someone like me, on a not very high income, part ownership is definitely a way of bridging the gap between renting and owning.

# At Home

Physically, my upper half is relatively OK and I try to keep myself fairly fit. Not having problems in the hips and shoulders means that I can do most things for myself around the flat, including bathing and dressing. A home help comes in twice a week to do heavy jobs like washing, ironing and cleaning. If it's a question of wiping surfaces clean, making sure the washing-up is done or clearing up the odd spillage, I do that myself. Friends help me do the shopping, but that's about all the help I need.

Gradually I have become more independent. In my last place, where there was a warden living in, I had to look after myself at the weekends, and get my own breakfasts, but on weekdays you could buy an evening meal if you wanted to. That is what I did for the first couple of years, then I began to find that the cooked meals were really too early in the evening for me. They served them from six to six-thirty, and I found I was wanting something more later on. By eleven o'clock I was making big rounds of cheese sandwiches, or toasting four crumpets. I began to put on weight, which is particularly bad for someone with arthritis because you want to put less stress on your joints, not more. One morning I took half an hour to get out of the bath, and I thought: this has got to stop. So I started to do a bit more on my own. I don't think I boiled an egg for myself until I was twenty-eight.

Now I am in the flat I have to look after myself all the time. On weekdays I have my main meal at work, thanks to a kind of Caribbean Meals-on-Wheels organization called the Pepperpot Club, which used to have an office downstairs from us. In the evenings mostly I make myself a snack – beans on toast and fruit, or fish fingers, or something like that.

At the weekends I try to cook proper meals. One of my specialities is spaghetti bolognese. I am getting into chilli, too, and there is a casserole dish which I like doing. I have a grill-up from time to time – that's like a fry-up without the hot fat spitting at you and it's more healthy! I have also developed a new tuna fish recipe [*laughter*]. In the oil of the tuna fish I fry onion, mushroom, garlic, perhaps some chilli powder, tomato purée and fresh tomatoes. I serve it with either rice or pasta, and add the tuna fish at the last minute.

I am getting better at looking after myself because I am more experienced at it and now feel able to try new things. I plan ahead very carefully, and buy in bulk whenever possible. I have a good circle of friends who are usually available to help me, and now the system only breaks down very occasionally – about once every two or three months – when I find I am desperate for money, for instance, but can't cash my Mobility Allowance because no-one is around to take me to the post office. At times like that I realize how dependent I am on other people. I don't worry about it very much; it's annoying on the day but it's not a blight on my life.

In my spare time I listen to music, play a bit of chess and do crosswords if someone is there to read out the clues. You can get braille crosswords but I find it takes too long to do the mechanical bits, so I prefer ordinary newspaper puzzles. I also read a lot of talking books.

I don't need any special aids in the flat for my arthritis, but I do label things like tins and music cassettes in braille, and the central heating controls are in braille, too. Around the flat my eyesight is my biggest problem; I am usually OK but I can still trip over a bin if I leave it sticking out slightly. Once I am outside, however, the arthritis is the biggest problem, because it limits my mobility, the kinds of transport I can use, and so on.

When I first came here I hoped I might be able to nip to the corner shop or the post office by myself. I could probably just about walk to the post office, but I doubt if I could get back. The pavement is very bad along here and I don't think my ankles could stand it; I think I would trip up. Even if it was a dead smooth run I would be nervous of going, because of the risk of being mugged. I have to face the fact that I am a very vulnerable target, so I would be worried all the time about being able to get home safely. I'd certainly have to stop in the pub on the way [*laughter*]!

# FROM STUDENT
# TO WORKER

## Judith Fitzgerald

---

Judith Fitzgerald has had rheumatoid arthritis since she was
seventeen, five years ago. Despite this she carried on with her
A levels, passed them, and got into university. She took her
degree in geography and now works for the Department of
Health and Social Security (DHSS) in Manchester. She
explains here how she managed to achieve all this.

---

I was healthy and had no trouble at all in my Lower Sixth year.
Then my wrists became sore and suddenly the arthritis flared
up during the summer holidays. I went back to school but was in
great pain and was referred to a specialist in Wrightington
Hospital, near my home in Darwen, Lancashire. From
November until April I was on bedrest, and only went home for
a fortnight at Christmas.

In the New Year I wanted to catch up with my A level work,
but the school was unhelpful and didn't want me to try. I
borrowed a friend's notes and carried on anyway, then with the
support of a hospital social worker I was allowed to continue. I
came out of hospital unable to walk much, but in May I was well
enough to take up driving again and I passed my test. It made all
the difference: I was able to get around and do things instead of
being stuck in one place.

In the summer I took my A levels. I got grade A in geography
and did well enough in two other subjects to take up a place at
Liverpool University. I went there in the autumn.

It was difficult at first, but I was given a small car which made
it much better. My knees were especially bad and walking was
often more than I could manage. I made some very good friends
who didn't mollycoddle me but who understood if I couldn't walk
somewhere. The hardest thing to explain to others is that with

arthritis you may feel well and able to get about one day, then the next you can hardly move at all. It was a help to be able to give my friends lifts in the car – everyone at university likes a lift!

During this time I was having gold injections, and every two weeks I had to have blood tests as well, which meant a 50 mile (80 km) drive because I wanted to be treated at my home hospital. Because of my studies and all the writing I had to do, my wrists swelled up and I had to take my first-year exams in the sick bay.

The time went by at Liverpool and I was very happy there. In the vacations, I would spend the first two weeks in hospital having injections into my joints. In the third year I began applying for jobs like everyone else. We all knew the job situation was bad and I thought that having arthritis would make it worse for me, but in July I got an offer of a job with the DHSS as an executive officer. I accepted, though it meant I needed to wait a year until the right vacancy arose in my area.

Looking back, I had to gear my job applications to something I could cope with physically, so obviously I could not put in for outdoor work. Some of my friends applied for jobs at the same places as I did, and there were times I felt I was being discriminated against, such as when they were asked to an interview and I wasn't. On the form we should all look the same, but there is usually a space where you are asked to say if you have any health problems. To me it is silly to put down 'I am disabled'. I don't feel disabled. What I liked about the Civil Service was that it didn't make any difference to them, and I am glad I took up their offer.

I share a house in Manchester with a friend from university who is working here as a teacher. In my job I get moved around the various sections and at the moment I am a visiting officer, going out to see people and talk to them, which I enjoy very much. My joints feel more worn, but I am more energetic now. Some days are bad, but I work on the principle of mind over matter. I have to have an aim in mind, and I have decided that going out to do something must help the joints. Well, it definitely helps mine.

# KEEPING BUSY

## INTRODUCTION

Having arthritis does not necessarily mean that you have to give up a favourite hobby. Nor does it mean that you cannot take up a new one. As Daphne Higginson demonstrates with her garden, success and satisfaction are well within reach – it's all a matter of planning and adapting to suit your own abilities.

## Craftwork and Other Pastimes

Whether you can participate in craftwork or not is mainly a question of movement. If you can keep your fingers mobile and nimble, you will be able to sew, do embroidery and many other crafts and hobbies. Even if you have difficulty in threading a needle, this need not be a problem for you can get a threading machine to do it for you, or use a self-threading needle. The important thing is to keep the skills you have going if you possibly can. They help to make life interesting: another project, another goal to aim at.

The choice of what to do is very wide. In her book *Healthy Living Over 55* Laura Mitchell lists sewing, knitting, carpentry, painting, flower arranging, collage work and baking. She adds, 'I know one gentleman who discovered the joys of bread making when he was over sixty. Making soft toys is another pleasurable occupation with a satisfying end product.' As for herself, she collects her old used stamps and postcards. 'I send them to The Stamp Officer, The Prison, Dartmoor, Devon. They tidy them up and sell them in aid of the Lifeboat Institution.'

Rosemary Sutcliff confesses to crazes: 'I am a typical Sagittarian. I have crazes which come and go. Usually they are the arty-crafty sort – collage, for instance, or crochet.

They may last for years, then they wear off and another one comes along.'

Did you know that men are good at embroidery? It is certainly nothing to be shy about. Laura Mitchell remembers a patient complaining to her that he found his home life boring. His wife watched television all the time and he did not want to do that. Was there something interesting that he could take up?

Laura suggested that he tried going down to the pub occasionally, to meet other people and have a chat. 'I can't,' he replied, 'I'm an alcoholic.'

It seemed he really was stuck. Then Laura had the idea of suggesting embroidery. The man was doubtful at first, but then, partly through desperation perhaps, he agreed to give it a try. He did, and soon was proudly showing off his new creations. For him, embroidery offered an entirely fresh channel for his thoughts and energies – and kept him out of mischief!

By the way, if you would like to try sewing or embroidery, but have trouble holding something still while you work on it, there is a special frame that you can buy. This can be fixed to a table or chair and leaves you free to concentrate on the main task.

The Disabled Living Foundation's Aids Centre has a permanent display which includes knitting and sewing aids, self-opening scissors, etc.

The following four chapters concentrate on two other areas of leisure: gardening and swimming. For a list of further ideas, organizations and books to read, see the 'Help' section at the end of the book.

# IN THE GARDEN

## Daphne Higginson

---

Daphne Higginson has had rheumatoid arthritis for sixteen years. Two years ago she had both her hips replaced, and more recently a knee joint. She also has arthritis in her hands, wrists and shoulders. Despite these limitations she decided to redesign the garden of her East Sussex home, where she lives with her mother, and now maintains it in immaculate order.

---

I looked at my weed-infested garden, at the mossy brick path and the paving stones I could never lift, and decided I had to start again from scratch. I had just come home from a spell in hospital. If I really wanted a garden that I would be able to plant and maintain more or less by myself, I would have to go back to basics, as though I were moving into a new house. I started to make a plan.

Too much grass would be difficult for me to maintain. I can stand for about ten minutes, but I dislike bending and cannot kneel down or lift anything heavy. I decided to have a fairly large patio area, keeping a smaller patch of grass which a neighbour would mow for me.

I would not be able to deal with borders in the ordinary way. I would need raised beds, high enough for me to sit on while I worked and narrow enough for me to reach across. I drew a plan of the garden and cut out some small pieces of card about ¾ in (2 cm) square. I coloured these to represent grass, earth or patio and pushed them about on the plan until I had achieved the kind of shapes I wanted and the right overall balance. I think curves are more interesting than straight lines, so I have given almost everything in the garden a curvy outline.

To do the initial heavy work of clearing the ground, 'rotavating' it, then building the patio and the raised beds, I obviously needed help. I had not long retired from teaching, because of my arthritis, and still had some money from that; so I decided to invest part of it in a new garden, and employed a local man experienced in landscaping to do the heavy work.

My plan would not suit everyone with arthritis. Someone capable of hoeing or digging, for instance, would be able to cope with ordinary flat borders. Grass, too, would not be such a problem to a gardener who could bend enough to mow it and trim the edges. A friend once suggested I get an electric trimmer to do the edges, but I can hardly lift one, let alone operate it.

'Going miniature' is another solution I have adopted. I would not be able to prune an ordinary rose bush; the stems are too thick. I do have miniature roses, however, and can prune them with a pair of scissors.

There is a forsythia which has survived from the old garden because it could not be dug out, and a neighbour comes and cuts that back for me. Friends helped me to put in two dwarf apple trees. I won't be able to prune them myself, but I know I can ask my friends to do it for me. One has to adapt to one's circumstances.

## Choosing Plants

Initially I chose my plants by looking at neighbours' gardens and seeing what grew well for them. We are not far from the sea here and have very high winds, so anything growing in the garden has to stand up to salt-laden gales. I am able to drive and I went round some garden centres, too. As well as liking the look of a plant, it is important for people with limited movement to know how big it will grow and whether it is likely to spread. Anything high or invasive is probably not a good idea. This has to be borne in mind in addition, of course, to the other considerations of soil, sun or shade, and so on. Never be in a hurry to stock a garden.

Along the south-facing side I have a small ground-level bed. I can cope with this from my gardening stool as long as the plants help me by spreading to keep down the weeds without themselves growing too large. I have a pulmonaria, thrift, a pink, a harebell which comes up and goes down in winter, and a tree peony which is sulking at the moment because it has just been moved, but it should grow quite large eventually. The thrift was transplanted from the front garden and is doing much better in its new site. I learn about these things as I go along. Aquilegias do well around here, too, so I have some in my garden. Against the fence are a climbing rose and a berberis. The rose will get too big for me to prune, but I wanted some plants to cover the bare fencing.

For the raised bed, as I have now discovered that you can get climbing miniature roses, I will be having at least one of those, and some more ordinary miniatures which I will put all along the bed. My other big future thing will be alpines. Among the other plants I already have are two potentillas, which grow very well here, a saxifrage, a miniature geranium, and a Christmas rose which I am encouraging to spread sideways. Against the fence is a cotoneaster, which was here before, and a clematis which is trained along a piece of trellis (my mother fixed this to the fence).

I keep one section of the garden for herbs. I have thyme, sage, parsley, camomile and feverfew, which is meant to be good for arthritis. (I have been eating the leaves for a while now, but it doesn't seem to have done me much good!)

In one corner I was going to have a wild garden, but I have gone off the idea. The wild flowers all look too much like weeds and if they were to spread I would be creating a lot of trouble for myself later on. There is a patch of bluebells which I want to take out. As I can't dig them out myself, I will probably wait until they come up next time and then get someone else to do it for me. A man who lives round the corner from me has already dug some out; he takes them down to the river bank to naturalize. When the bluebells have finally gone, I will put in some more plants.

And so we go on. It is all taking shape – but it does take time, especially when you have arthritis. However, gardening has become a way of life for me, so I accept that I must be patient.

# In the Toolshed

On the whole, gardening centres do not cater for people with arthritis. It depends which sort of arthritis you have, but in my case I find that most of the factory-made tools they stock are too heavy – so I make some of my own.

My weeding tool is a carving fork attached to a light broom handle. It works very well and it means I don't have to bend. I have a little spade which is really a long-handled trowel, and I can use that for some tasks. I also have a lot of my father's old forks and spades, which are very good but not for me, as I can't lever and lift properly.

To apply weedkiller, I use a plastic container (an old syrup pot) with three holes near the top through which I have threaded some string to make a handle. I put the weedkiller in the container, which I lower to the ground by the string, then I dip a brush into it (a paint brush with a long handle) and paint the weedkiller on to the area being dealt with.

I have a bulb planter which works on roughly similar lines. It is an old peach can with the ends removed. At one end is a string handle, fixed through holes near the top of the can. I place the can on the ground, press it in with my foot, then pull it out with the string, and that leaves me a hole big enough for a small bulb.

I use my planter in partnership with a device I saw on television. It's a piece of plastic pipe, which is used as a chute to slide the bulb, or whatever, down to its planting position. That way you don't need to bend, and if the bulb lands the wrong way up you can poke it into place with a 'helping hand'.

For watering, I keep a hose permanently out in the garden. If I get tired of holding the hose, I have a piece of plastic guttering with a short length of downpipe attached. I put the hose through the pipe and then stand the guttering on its end, to serve as a support; the hose can be wedged with a stone to stop it jumping. For local watering in small quantities I use an old teapot.

# TRY SWIMMING

Swimming – which for our purposes means exercising in warm water – can be marvellously beneficial to people with arthritis. Water lifts our gravity from us as we float. Pains disappear, and within minutes the disabled are astonished to find that they can hold their own, even compete, with their able-bodied friends.

'We look for ability, not disability,' says Dr Joan Martin. She is the chief instructor of Kensington Emperors, one of 130 clubs belonging to the Association for Swimming Therapy. Each Friday evening, from seven to nine o'clock, up to eighty members gather at Kensington Sports Centre in Walmer Road, West London.

'We have every possible disability amongst our members,' says Dr Martin, 'and every age from five to seventy-five. People with arthritis find that the water gives them relief from pain, and the buoyancy allows them to move stiff joints more freely than they can manage out of the pool. The temperature of the water can be a worry, but modern public pools usually keep to a standard level of more than 80°F (27°C) and that is OK for most people. If it is much hotter, people find it uncomfortable and then they don't want to stay.

'We teach everyone on a one-to-one basis. Non-swimmers stay in the pool for twenty minutes, and swimmers go into the deep water with their instructors. They can stay in the pool for the full two hours if they want to.'

For further information about the Association, and details of a branch near you, contact Bill Wood, The Secretary, Treetops, Swan Hill, Ellesmere, Salop SY12 0LZ.

In the following pages, two Emperors and a sports presenter talk about how swimming has helped with their arthritis.

# AT HOME IN WATER

## Joan Harris

Joan Harris has osteoarthritis which affects almost all her joints. She spent her working life as a secretary in the legal profession, getting around as best she could, and has gained a lot from her time at the swimming club, which she joined in the early sixties.

I had rheumatism when I was very young. My mother used to take me to the Children's Hospital in Tite Street, London. I had a TB hip and in my teens I had a lot of tests and x-rays. When I went home they said, 'Tell her it's only arthritis.'

I got myself a job and carried on working into my thirties. Then my mother had a stroke and I had to keep going to earn a living and look after the home as well.

I always wanted to swim, but my mother – partly because of my disability – was very nervy about it and didn't want me to try. When she died, I decided: 'Right, I'm *going* to swim.' At first I didn't go to a handicapped club – I went to the YMCA, as they had a pool there. Old Reg Brickett, the former champion, was teaching children to swim and I asked him if he'd teach me. 'Yes,' he said. 'Come next Saturday.'

I went, and a young woman took me and gave me lessons. In the fourth lesson I did a width. Then I learnt to float. I decided to look around for a handicapped club that I could join, and in the end I found out about the Kensington Emperors.

I went there and I was well away. I did ⅔ mile (1000 m) one night. I swim on my back; if I turn on my face, I find the force of the water hurts my old hip. It's like walking on a broken bone so I try not to move it too much. I find no difficulty in floating: I get in the water and lift up my legs and lie there. It frightens me that I could go to sleep! It's really like lying on a very soft bed. Once you are in the water and haven't got any weight you can move so much more. I find I get great joy from it.

# FEELING SO
# MUCH BETTER

## Margaret Joel

---

Margaret Joel began to suffer from rheumatoid arthritis
thirteen years ago, when she was fifty-nine. Several years
went by before she heard about the Kensington Emperors, but
once she started going to the pool it changed her whole
outlook.

---

The arthritis took time to get where it is. It's all over the place
now, but when it began it was just in the elbow. After that it
appeared in the feet. Then it went into the knee, then into the
shoulder. Gradually it went all the way round.

I first heard about the swimming club from a lady at my
branch of Arthritis Care. At the time a hydrotherapy pool was
being built at my local hospital, St Stephen's, but it wasn't quite
ready. I said to her, 'I hope I'll get my name down for that. It'll
do me good.' I wasn't a water person. I couldn't say I'd been
swimming all my life, but I felt it would help me. You clutch at
straws. She said, 'You don't have to wait for that. You can join
this club in North Kensington.'

My husband went to the Town Hall and got a form. I went to
the doctor to make sure my heart was all right. He said it was, so
I went to the club. It altered my whole performance altogether.
Before then I hadn't been to my Arthritis Care branch meetings
for about two years because I couldn't get about much, as I had
to be in a wheelchair. But at the swimming club I was mixing
with people again. I liked it. I hadn't swum before. In fact, I
hadn't been in the water since I left school, and that was when I
was fourteen.

They put me in the water and made me feel so much a part of
them. I got on all right with the swimming. I didn't think I would.
It was all right once I got over the embarrassment and stopped

thinking: all these young people, now what am I going to do? I felt a bit silly. But they were so kind, and Dr Martin helped me, and *she* wasn't particularly young. Even the escort who looked after us in the ambulance – they pick you up from home and bring you back again – was sixty-eight so I didn't feel quite so bad. Then we picked up a lady who was eighty, so I didn't feel out of it at all after that.

I really enjoyed the swimming and looked forward to the Friday nights. It did my morale a lot of good. I hadn't seen so many disabled people before and they coped with it very nicely. I thought, well, if they can do it, so can I.

I felt so much better that I thought I would soon be able to manage without the wheelchair. Then I had an operation on my knee, and that was a success. When the time came to get out of bed in the hospital, I had no trouble getting up on my feet again. Because of the swimming the muscles around the knee were much stronger than those of the other patients. Even the nurses remarked how supple I was. The surgeon was thrilled, because I could walk with just one stick after three days.

For the next twelve months I went along fine. I could do my bits here at home and every Friday I went swimming. Perhaps I got careless and didn't look out enough, because one day I came back to the house, didn't take as much care as I should have done, fell over and broke my hip.

I got over that, and in time I went back to the swimming. But then the arthritis seemed to go all over the place. The tendons snapped in one hand, and then the other knee went. I had the hand put right, but the doctors said that all these operations were not good for my heart, and I have had to stay indoors since, except for going to the hospital.

It's sad. I can't wait to get back to swimming. It's the only exercise I know where you can move about and not get any pain. Trouble is, as you get older it takes longer to get over things. The arthritis is all over me and now I also have fluid on the knee and it's got quite swollen. But perhaps I'll be able to start swimming again one day.

# A LATE STARTER

## David Icke

Television sports presenter David Icke has only recently
learned to swim – and wishes he had conquered his fears
much sooner.

When I was a little nipper I went paddling in the sea at Caister,
in Norfolk. I tripped up, went under, and all through my
childhood I was frightened to death of water. Even when we
moved to the Isle of Wight two years ago I could not swim a
stroke. The fear of water was still with me.

This time I decided to deal with it. I had lessons and learned to
swim. Now I am a complete convert. From the point of view of
my arthritis I think swimming is fantastically good. The
movement is smooth, there is no jerkiness; you can support
yourself in the water without having to battle against the usual
element – air; and it is wonderful for loosening up stiff joints.

It is also a great way to stay fit. Since my arthritis became so
bad that I had to give up football, I have found it very difficult to
take on any form of physical exercise. Swimming, however, is
something I can do.

I swim nearly every day in the local baths. I do at least ten
lengths of breaststroke, which is the easiest stroke for me. I can
go at my own pace and it sets me up to fight the stresses of
arthritis. The fitter you are, the better you will feel.

# LONELY TIMES

## INTRODUCTION

It is no secret that having arthritis can make people depressed. It is an extra burden, especially difficult to bear when there is little or no relief from pain, or a daunting operation is in prospect, or the right person is not available to share the sufferer's thoughts.

The contributions that follow are all from people who have talked about their arthritis in previous chapters. We hope that these further thoughts and revelations may give hope when it is needed.

# BY MYSELF,
# BUT NOT ALONE

## Alice Pearl

People talk about feeling lonely. Although I live by myself I never, ever, feel alone. Since I was a child I have been conscious that Someone is there with me. When I am in difficulty, it gives me great inner strength. Then something happens, which *proves* that my instinct is right. I will tell you about one of those times.

Two years ago, I had been out to a branch meeting of Arthritis Care. I came home at about ten o'clock and my nurse got me into bed and settled. That night my daughter Betty drove back to Nottingham from Edinburgh, where she had been working. When she got to her house she rang me, as she always does, night and morning, to see how I was.

'Are you all right, Mummy?'

'Yes,' I told her, I was all right. The nurse had been and I was in bed. I said goodnight to Betty and put the phone down.

Some minutes later I realized that there was an obstacle at the foot of my bed. I thought to myself: 'That could be a hazard in the morning.' I decided I had better put things right there and then.

I brought myself down to floor level on my electric bed. All of a sudden I slipped sideways and fell flat on the floor. It was eleven o'clock at night. I couldn't get up. I shivered at the thought of what had just happened to me, and what it meant.

'Betty won't ring me now,' I told myself. Nobody would be coming in until nine o'clock in the morning. What was I going to do?

I had hurt my back in the fall. I was cold and uncomfortable, quite apart from the pain. After a few minutes I got hold of my stick, crawled to the window and knocked on it. I knocked for some while, off and on, but nobody was about at that time of night. I tried to reach the telephone, up on its shelf. I pulled at it with my stick but all that came down was the receiver. The rest stayed where it was, and I could not shift it without the risk of catching the wires of the electric kettle and bringing that down on top of me. Too dangerous. No, I mustn't do that. I sat back. What *was* I going to do?

I tried to think positively. What were my advantages? I'd got a light on – thank God for that. A blanket had come down with me and I wrapped myself in it. I tried to get comfortable and settle, but I could not sleep. Midnight came and went. One o'clock. Two o'clock. Still no sleep. I was intensely worried about getting pneumonia, stuck there on my bottom on the floor, but there was nothing I could do, and I had all but given up hope, when suddenly the door opened – and in walked Betty!

'Good heavens!' she cried. She stared at me in horror, then immediately rang for an ambulance. She was in a very emotional state as she listened while I told her what had happened. Then she told me her side of the story, which was even more astounding.

At midnight, after her long drive from Edinburgh, she had gone to bed, taken two sleeping tablets and switched off the light. At a quarter past two something made her wake up with a jolt. 'Mummy's in trouble!' she said to herself, there in the dark of her bedroom. She *knew*.

She picked up the phone and dialled my number. Engaged. That settled it. She must be right. She threw a coat over her pyjamas and rushed down to her car. She drove here at full speed, through red lights and everything. When she stopped outside and saw my light was on, her heart sank. She thought I'd been mugged! She let herself in, bless her, and there I sat.

What more proof could there be that Someone is with me and looks after me? I said to Betty, 'It's true! I'll never be afraid again!'

I can only see the events of that night in one way. I had struggled and tried to do everything I could for myself. I made myself as comfortable as I could on that floor, but then there was nothing else I could do – and it wasn't enough. If I had remained there until nine o'clock, I am sure I would not have survived. I reckon it was at the very moment I ran out of things to do for myself that the Lord took over.

'Come on, Betty,' He said to my sleeping daughter. 'Wake up. She needs you.'

# BEFORE THE
# OPERATION

## Alan Rogers

The hip operation is heavy, messy, intimidating. In the operating theatre there are mallets, spikes and all kinds of fearsome implements. Several people had already told me that they virtually take your leg off to do the operation.

When the time came to face up to all that, I was glad that I had the strength of my religious beliefs to support me. In the week beforehand I prayed a lot, and I knew that my friends at church were praying for me, too. I was able to reach a stage where I felt I was in God's hands. On the day itself, I felt almost peaceful.

I was prepared to accept whatever might happen, but I also felt more hopeful. I believe that God heals through clever doctors and nurses as well as through miracles. The fact that I was in the hands of highly competent medical professionals made a world of difference and helped me to approach the whole thing with optimism. At the same time I felt that God was looking after me, so even if the doctors got it wrong, I would still be all right!

# BETTER WHEN THE SUN SHINES

## Tony Van den Bergh

When I began work as a freelance reporter for the BBC, the equipment we had to carry was heavy and awkward. I found I could carry it all right – and for considerable distances – but the result was always the same: pain afterwards. This was partly, I am sure, because the adrenaline had stopped flowing. I am convinced that arthritic pain is tremendously subject to a person's varying moods.

If the pain is bad, it is all too easy to make yourself miserable. At one time I lived by the Thames at Bray in Berkshire. I was preparing a radio programme on arthritis and a lot of people wrote to me saying I shouldn't be living so close to a river as it could only make my arthritis worse. I asked several leading consultants about this and they all said the same thing: 'How can dampness in the atmosphere affect what goes on inside your joints?'

I thought about this and decided they must be right. But, I also thought, you have to consider the mental side as well. If, for example, there is a fog on the river and everything is grey and bleak, you are bound to feel a bit miserable and this reminds you of your pain, which then starts to hurt more than usual. However, when it is sunny and bright, the riverside is one of the most beautiful places you could possibly be. The views are marvellous, the sun warms you through, you put your shoulders back and feel terrific. No trace of pain at all.

# KEEPING A BALANCE

## Phil Smith

People with arthritis have their problems, but I find it doesn't help me to think about mine too much. If I let my thoughts wander on in an uncontrolled way, they would quickly get me down.

The next time you find yourself having negative thoughts, try to counter them with some positive ones. For instance, I could give you a whole list of things I can't do or find extremely difficult:

I can't jog.

I can't prepare vegetables.

I can't sit on the floor and get up again.

I can't scratch my back or scrub it.

When I feel bad, I can't even wash myself.

I could go on. The point is, if I thought about all the negative things all the time, I'd end up never getting out of bed.

My way out, if I'm feeling gloomy, is to think of all the things I *can* do:

I'm going up to London tomorrow.

I went swimming on my holidays.

Not all that long ago I went on a scooter – I never thought I'd do that again.

I went rock climbing and abseiling last year.

These thoughts, and sometimes the memories that go with them, are very important to me. They help me to switch off the bad days and focus on the good days.

In any case, 'I can't' is never the end of the story. If the problem is about something you are unable to do, try asking someone else to do it for you, someone in your family, perhaps, or a friend. If that is not the answer, ask yourself if this something you can't do is really so important after all; perhaps you will find it is not, in which case you need not bother yourself about it in future. And even if it does need to be done, don't worry. There is always a way of adapting your approach so you get round the problem in the end. Always.

# HELP

## (Is never far away)

## ARTHRITIS CARE

This book was conceived by Arthritis Care, the charity whose official aims are:

'To help arthritis and rheumatism sufferers with information, advice and practical aid and to strive for improved facilities for those afflicted by the rheumatic diseases.'

Arthritis Care has more than 40,000 members and an extensive regional network with nearly 400 branches. It was founded in 1947 by Arthur Mainwaring Bowen, then a twenty-five-year-old sufferer from ankylosing spondylitis (spinal arthritis), and was formerly known as The British Rheumatism & Arthritis Association. It is a self-help organization, and many members find it useful to belong to one of the branches and enjoy the social and morale-boosting benefits of regular meetings, outings and a chance to talk over their problems in an understanding atmosphere. Others prefer just to belong to the organization, receiving the quarterly newspaper, *Arthritis News*, and other information about Arthritis Care's activities. The association maintains a Welfare Department which answers thousands of inquiries every year. There is also a Home Visiting Service for housebound members, a residential home for the severely disabled, four holiday centres offering specially adapted hotel accommodation, and ten specially adapted self-catering units for family holidays.

For younger members there is a very active 35 Group, which publishes its own magazine, *In Contact*, and has a regional network.

The Lupus Group helps people suffering from systemic lupus erythematosus (SLE). Currently it has eighteen regional branches and also publishes its own magazine, *News and Views*.

Arthritis Care is also associated with The Lady Hoare Trust, which looks after the welfare of children who are sufferers, offering support to children and their parents.

For further information about Arthritis Care, and details of membership, please write to:
Arthritis Care, 6 Grosvenor Crescent, London SW1X 7ER; tel. 01-235 0902

## Other Organizations to Contact

**The Arthritis & Rheumatism Council**, 41 Eagle Street, London WC1R 4AR; tel. 01-405 8572
The Council raises funds for research into rheumatic diseases. It publishes many useful medical booklets and leaflets (see 'Books to Read', page 156), and its own magazine.

**Disability Alliance**, 25 Denmark Street, London WC2H 8NJ; tel. 01-240 0806
A national federation of organizations supporting the disabled. Its Educational and Research Association publishes *Disability Rights Handbook*, a large-format paperback with detailed, easy-to-understand information on a comprehensive range of matters of interest to the disabled. This is the book to consult about grants, benefits, problems with housing, mobility, children, money matters and much else. The latest edition is available from the above address, price £3.00 post free.

**National Ankylosing Spondylitis Association**, 6 Grosvenor Crescent, London SW1X 7ER; tel. 01-235 9585
A charity providing information about ankylosing spondylitis, including specialist advice on social problems. It publishes a guide book, and members receive a twice-yearly bulletin.

**RADAR, Royal Association for Disability and Rehabilitation**, 25 Mortimer Street, London W1N 8AB; tel. 01-637 5400
A co-ordinating body for physical disability which publishes material on a variety of topics concerning the disabled. RADAR is a regular sponsor of the annual NAIDEX exhibition of aids and equipment for the disabled.

# HOME AIDS

## Disabled Living Foundation

This is a charitable trust concerned with helping disabled people of any age to adapt their daily lives to their particular disability. Its Aids Centre, the first of its kind in the world, offers a comprehensive standing exhibition of aids to help in all aspects of daily life (see pages 26, 33, 37 and 78). Professional health workers take patients and clients there to see and try out equipment, and disabled people and their relatives are especially welcome. The aids are not for sale but information about suppliers and prices can be provided. All visitors must make an appointment in advance. Contact: Disabled Living Foundation, 380–384 Harrow Road, London W9 2HU; tel. 01-289 6111.

The DLF also offers specialist advice on clothing, incontinence, music, physical recreation and visual handicap, and publishes a number of books about the daily living problems of disabled people.

Aids may also be seen at the following regional centres. As with London, contact the centre before visiting; an appointment is usually necessary. Check that the centre can deal with your requirements.

## Aids Centres Offering a Fully Comprehensive Service

| | |
|---|---|
| BELFAST | Prosthetic, Orthotic & Aids Service, Musgrave Park Hospital, Stockman's Lane, Belfast BT9 7JB; tel. 0232 669501 |
| BIRMINGHAM | Disabled Living Centre, 260 Broad Street, Birmingham, W. Midlands B1 2HF; tel. 021-643 0980 |
| CAERPHILLY | Aids and Information Centre, Wales Council for the Disabled, Caerbragdy Industrial Estate, Bedwas Road, Caerphilly, Mid-Glamorgan CF8 3SL; tel. 0222 887325/6/7 |
| EDINBURGH | Lothian Disabled Living Centre, Astley Ainslie Hospital, Grange Loan, Edinburgh EH9 2HL; tel. 031-447 6271, ext. 241 |
| LEEDS | The William Merritt Disabled Living Centre, St Mary's Hospital, Greenhill Road, Leeds, W. Yorkshire LS12 3QE; tel. 0532 793140 |

| | |
|---|---|
| LEICESTER | TRAIDS (Trent Region Aids, Information and Demonstration Service), 76 Clarendon Park Road, Leicester LE2 3AD; tel. 0533 700747/8 |
| LIVERPOOL | Merseyside Aids Centre, Youens Way, East Prescot Road, Liverpool L14 2EP; tel. 051-228 9221 |
| MANCHESTER | Disabled Living Services, Disabled Living Centre, Redbank House, 4 St Chad's Street, Cheetham, Manchester M8 8QA; tel. 061-832 3678 |
| NEWCASTLE-UPON-TYNE | Newcastle-upon-Tyne Council for the Disabled, The Dene Centre, Castles Farm Road, Newcastle-upon-Tyne, Tyne & Wear NE3 1PH; tel. 091 2840480 |
| SHEFFIELD | Sheffield Independent Living Centre, 108 The Moor, Sheffield, S. Yorkshire S1 4PD; tel. 0742 737025 |
| SOUTHAMPTON | Southampton Aid & Equipment Centre, Southampton General Hospital, Tremona Road, Southampton, Hampshire SO9 4XY; tel. 0703 777222, ext. 3414/3233 |
| STOCKPORT | Aids/Assessment Unit, Stockport Area Health Authority, St Thomas's Hospital, Shawheath, Stockport, Greater Manchester; tel. 061-483 1010, ext. 15 |
| SWINDON | The Swindon Centre for Disabled Living, The Hawthorn Centre, Cricklade Road, Swindon, Wiltshire SN2 1AF; tel. 0793 643966 |

# Aids Centres Offering a Limited Service

| | |
|---|---|
| BLACKPOOL | Disabled Living Centre, 8 Queen Street, Blackpool, Lancashire FY1 1PD; tel. 0253 21084, ext. 1 |
| DUDLEY | Dudley Aids & Assessment Centre, 1 St Giles Street, Netherton, Dudley, W. Midlands; tel. 0384 55433 |
| PAISLEY | Disability Centre for Independent Living, Community Services Centre, Queen's Street, Paisley, Strathclyde; tel. 041-887 0597 |

PORTSMOUTH          Disabled Living Centre, Prince Albert Road,
                    Eastney, Portsmouth, Hampshire PO4 9HR;
                    tel. 0705 737174

These lists are correct at the time of going to press; up-to-date
details can be obtained from the DLF.

Other places where aids and equipment may be seen include local
Occupational Therapy departments in hospitals and local Social
Services departments; some of the latter have assessment centres.

In Scotland a travelling exhibition of aids tours the country. For
details, contact:
Scottish Council on Disability, Princes House, 5 Shandwick Place,
Edinburgh EH2 4RG; tel. 031-229 8632

# TRANSPORT AIDS

The best general source for advice about transport is *Door to Door*, a
free guide published by the Department of Transport (see page 60 for
the list of contents). To obtain a copy, write (no stamp needed) to:
Department of Transport and Environment, *Door to Door* Guide,
FREEPOST, Victoria Road, South Ruislip, Middlesex HA4 0NZ

Access to public buildings is a problem for many people with
arthritis. RADAR produce a series of local access guides, of which
forty to fifty are usually in print at any one time. For information
about these and other publications, contact:
RADAR, Royal Association for Disability and Rehabilitation,
25 Mortimer Street, London W1N 8AB; tel. 01-637 5400

For advice about rail travel and fare concessions, ask at your local
British Rail station or write to:
British Railways Board (Central Publicity Unit), Mulberry House,
Marylebone, London NW1

For Londoners, or people visiting London, wanting to travel by
underground, there is a useful guide for elderly and disabled
passengers called *Access to the Underground*. For a copy, write to:
Unit for Disabled Passengers, London Regional Transport,
55 Broadway, London SW1H 0BD

For people new to wheelchairs, including those who push them, the
British Red Cross Society publishes a booklet, *People in
Wheelchairs*, price 43p inc. p & p. For a copy, write to:
Supply Dept, British Red Cross Society, 4 Grosvenor Crescent,
London SW1X 7EQ

# Cars and Driving

These organizations offer help with a range of motoring problems:

**Assistance and Independence for Disabled People (AID)**,
182 Brighton Road, Coulsdon, Surrey CR3 2NF; tel. 01-645 9014
A commercial company with a range of fifty cars available for hire-purchase on a no-deposit basis.

**Banstead Place Mobility Centre**, Park Road, Banstead, Surrey SM7 3EE; tel. 073-73 51674
An advisory service on the different types of vehicle available for disabled people. Also has a multi-discipline assessment service.

**Disabled Drivers' Association**, Ashwellthorpe Hall, Ashwellthorpe, Norwich, Norfolk NR6 1EX; tel. 050-841 449. Also at: 18 Creekside, London SE8 3DZ; tel. 01-692 7141
Self-help organization which works for independence through mobility.

**Disabled Drivers' Motor Club**, 1A Dudley Gardens, Ealing, London WI3 9LU; tel. 01-840 1515
Provides advice to its members on mobility problems, conversions, insurance discounts, etc.

**Disabled Living Foundation**, 380–384 Harrow Road, London W9 2HU; tel. 01-289 6111. In Scotland: **Scottish Council on Disability**, Princess House, 5 Shandwick Place, Edinburgh EH2 4RG; tel. 031-229 8632
Issues an annually updated information sheet on transport. This contains a list of firms specializing in conversion and adaptation work on cars. Other advice is available on car design, costs, and where to obtain adapted cars.

**Mobility Advice & Vehicle Information Service (MAVIS)**, Department of Transport, Transport and Road Research Laboratory, Crowthorne, Berkshire RG11 6AU; tel. 0344 779014
Offers personal assessment and practical advice on driving ability and car adaptations, and information on all aspects of transport (public and private) and outdoor mobility for people with disabilities.

**Mobility Information Service, MOTEC**, Unit 2a, Atcham Estate, Upton Magna, Shrewsbury, Salop SY4 4UG; tel. 074377 489
Voluntary organization able to provide information on cars, adaptations, costs, etc. Also issues leaflets covering all aspects of choosing, buying and converting a car. Personal assessment possible within 100 mile (160 km) radius of Shrewsbury.

**Motability**, Boundary House, 91–93 Charterhouse Street, London EC1M 6BT; tel. 01-253 1211
Voluntary organization set up to help people with disabilities to use their Mobility Allowance to buy or lease a car. Under their hire-purchase scheme it is also possible to buy an electric wheelchair.

**Steering Developments Ltd**, Unit 3, Eastman Way, Hemel
Hempstead, Herts HP2 7HF; tel. 0442 212918/9
Specialist commercial firm offering car conversions and
adaptations.

# HOBBIES AND PASTIMES

## Craftwork

For people wanting to take up a new handicraft, there are many
possibilities. Arthritis Care has a Homework Division, which
encourages housebound members to resume or develop a new
handicraft, such as toymaking, crochet or basketmaking. Local day
centres often provide opportunities for craftwork. If you are
interested in taking a part-time or full-time course, contact your
local education authority. The Women's Institute is also a good
source of information and encouragement. For a list of craft centres,
contact:
The Arts Council, 105 Piccadilly, London W1V 0AU; tel. 01-629 9495

## Gardening

Readers may like to join Horticultural Therapy, a charity which
helps elderly and handicapped gardeners. Members can receive
advice and practical help with their gardening problems, exchange
ideas, use the charity's library and information services, and receive
a quarterly magazine, *Growth Point*. For details, contact:
Horticultural Therapy, Goulds Ground, Vallis Way, Frome,
Somerset BA11 3DW; tel. 0373 64782

## Reading

There are two talking book services for people who find ordinary
books either difficult or impossible to manage. Both have an annual
subscription scheme. For further information, contact:
Royal National Institute for the Blind, Talking Book Service, Mount
Pleasant, Wembley, Middlesex HA0 1RR; tel. 01-903 6666

Talking Books for the Handicapped, National Listening Library, 12
Lant Street, London SE1 1QH; tel. 01-407 9417

## Swimming

The Association of Swimming Therapy has 130 member clubs in the
UK. For further information, contact:
Bill Wood, The Secretary, Association of Swimming Therapy,
Treetops, Swan Hill, Ellesmere, Salop SY12 0LZ; tel. 069-171 3542

The National Association of Swimming Clubs for the Handicapped has about 80 member clubs. It publishes a register of all disabled clubs and groups in the UK (more than 600 in all). To obtain a copy, contact:
National Association of Swimming Clubs for the Handicapped, 219 Preston Drove, Brighton, E. Sussex BN1 6FL; tel. 0273 559470

# BOOKS TO READ

## Clothes & Dressing

Ruston, Rosemary, *Dressing for Disabled People* (Disabled Living Foundation); available from DLF (Sales) Ltd, Book House, 45 East Hill, Wandsworth, London SW18 2QZ, price £3 inc. p & p.

Turnbull, Peggy, and Ruston, Rosemary, *Clothes Sense – for disabled people of all ages* (Piel-Caru for Disabled Living Foundation); available from DLF (Sales) Ltd, as above, price £9 inc.

## Cookery & Kitchen

Foott, S., and others, *Kitchen Sense for Disabled People* (DLF); available from DLF (Sales) Ltd, as above, price £9.45 inc. p & p.

Macfarlane, Ann, *Are You Cooking Comfortably?* (Arthritis Care); available from bookshops or from the distributors: Biblios, Glenside Industrial Estate, Partridge Green, Horsham, W. Sussex RH13 8LD, price £2.95 inc. p & p.

## Gardening

Cloet, Audrey, and Underhill, Chris, *Gardening Is for Everyone* (Souvenir Press)

Pays, Isobel, *Gardening in Retirement* (Age Concern); available from Age Concern at Bernard Sunley House, 60 Pitcairn Road, Mitcham, Surrey CR4 3LL, price £1.95 inc. p & p.

## General and Medical

Arthritis & Rheumatism Council booklets and leaflets; current booklets include: *Introducing Arthritis*, *Rheumatoid Arthritis Explained*, *Osteoarthritis Explained*, *Are You Sitting Comfortably?* (a guide to choosing easy chairs), *Your Home and Your Rheumatism*, *Ankylosing Spondylitis*, *Backache*, *Pain in the Neck*, *When Your Child Has Arthritis*, *Gout*, *Lupus (SLE)*, *Marriage, Sex and Arthritis*; current leaflets advise on *Tennis Elbow*, *Polymyalgia Rheumatica*, *A New Hip Joint*.

All are available free of charge from ARC, 41 Eagle Street, London WC1R 4AR. Please write enclosing a large s.a.e.

Darnborough, Ann, and Kinrade, Derek, *Directory of Aids for Disabled and Elderly People* (Woodhead Faulkner, Publishers, Ltd); available from booksellers at £14.95 or direct from the publishers at 32 Trumpington Street, Cambridge CB2 1QY, price £16.55 inc. p & p.

Disability Alliance, *Disability Rights Handbook*; current annual edition available from Publications, Disability Alliance, 25 Denmark Street, London WC2H 8NJ, price £3.00 post free.

Hart, Dr Frank Dudley, *Overcoming Arthritis* (Martin Dunitz)
Hughes, Dr Graham, *Lupus – a Guide for Patients* (booklet); available from Lupus Group, 6 Grosvenor Crescent, London SW1X 7ER, price £1
Jayson, Michael N., and Dixon, Allan St J., *Rheumatism and Arthritis* (Pan Books)
Lorig, Kate, and Fries, James F., *The Arthritis Helpbook* (Souvenir Press)
Mitchell, Laura, *Healthy Living Over 55 – The 'Getting On' Guide* (John Murray, Central Independent Television); *Simple Relaxation* (John Murray); *Simple Movement* (John Murray)
Phillips, Robert H., *Coping with Lupus* (Avery Press, Wayne, New Jersey); available from Lupus Group, 6 Grosvenor Crescent, London SW1X 7ER, price £5
Scott, J. T., *Arthritis & Rheumatism – The Facts* (Oxford University Press)
Unsworth, Heather, *Coping with Rheumatoid Arthritis* (Chambers)

## Personal Accounts

Joseph, Marie, *One Step at a Time* (Heinemann/Arrow)
La Fane, Pamela, *It's a Lovely Day, Outside* (Gollancz)
Pearl, Alice, *No Leg to Stand On* (available from the author at 11 Averton Square, Wollaton Park, Nottingham NG8 1AN)
Sutcliff, Rosemary, *Blue Remembered Hills – A Recollection* (Oxford University Press)

## Transport

Darnborough, Ann, and Kinrade, Derek, *Motoring and Mobility for Disabled People* (RADAR); available from RADAR at 25 Mortimer Street, London W1N 8AB, price £4 inc. p & p.

Department of Transport, *Ins and Outs of Car Choice – a guide for elderly and disabled people*; available from Department of Transport and Environment, Publications Sales Unit, Building 1, Victoria Road, South Ruislip, Middlesex HA4 0NZ, price £1.45 post free.

# INDEX